Presenting at Medical Meetings

Jim A. Reekers

Presenting at Medical Meetings

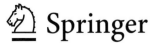 Springer

Prof. Dr. Jim A. Reekers
University of Amsterdam
Academic Medical Center
Department of Radiology
Meibergdreef 9
1105 AZ Amsterdam
The Netherlands
j.a.reekers@amc.uva.nl

ISBN: 978-3-642-12407-5   e-ISBN: 978-3-642-12408-2

DOI: 10.1007/978-3-642-12408-2

Springer Heidelberg Dordrecht London New York

Library of Congress Control Number: 2010931839

Cover design: eStudio Calamar, Figueres/Berlin

Printed on acid-free paper

Springer is part of Springer Science+Business Media (www.springer.com)

To Liesbeth den Besten, my wife, who opened my mind to see that you can only give a great lecture after careful and conscientious preparation.

Preface

Going to a medical meeting is a huge investment in terms of both time and money. There can be many reasons to go to a medical meeting: one could go as a participant attending the lectures, a presenter of a scientific abstract, an invited speaker, or even a keynote speaker. Although each of these groups has different goals and objectives, it is important for all to see that during the meeting their goals and objectives are met. Clearly flying 12 h to a medical meeting to give a 10-min scientific presentation that is poorly prepared and uses confusing slides has very little positive impact. It is not only a waste of time and money, but also an unjustifiable environmental burden.

There are many tips, tricks and simple rules that can help and guide you through a successful medical meeting. Presenting at a meeting is not, as many seem to think, a "natural talent", it is an art which can be learned. But it does require that you know about the basic rules and that you are willing and open for a reset. Forget about how you have been presenting in the past and start working on your new communication tools. You will be amazed about yourself. Many of the topics discussed in this book might seem obvious, but every time I go to a meeting I see the same mistakes again and again. Even renowned speakers who are more or less part of the inventory of every medical meeting can be seen making beginners' mistakes.

Small details, like which tie to wear, can have an impact on the audience's appreciation of your presentation. The biggest mistake a speaker can make is to have disorganised slides and a 20 min presentation when there is only 10-min speaking time available. This will all be discussed and illustrated with examples, that come mostly from my own long experience of the many medical meetings I have attended all over the world.

This book is not only based on my own personal view and experiences - most of what is discussed here can be found in literature on training sales managers, where good and clear communication is a vital element to success and survival. It is not a scientific book, so do not look for the level 1 evidence; justification for most of the content is my personal annoyance at yet another poor lecture. I have tried to write a book that is applicable to everybody, both novices and old meeting dinosaurs; a book that I still would like to read myself. I have therefore written it in a light tone, with many personal anecdotes, to make it more accessible. Although humour can be a powerful vehicle to carry a serious message, like all things in life, moderation is the key.

Although many parts of the book don't have the dry and serious approach of medical teaching books, the content has, first and foremost, an educational purpose.

It has always struck me that every medical meeting from every medical speciality all over the world is basically just the same; the same social structure, the same rules and the same challenges, differentiated only by the specialised presentation topics. I therefore also included a last chapter with some basic medical meeting information including the "social" environment of medical meetings. If you do not understand the medical meeting biotope of a meeting, your lectures will not be absorbed by your audience. This is therefore a book suitable for any physician going to a medical meeting, regardless of their speciality.

I hope that after reading this book you will have all the tools and basic requirements to become a professional presenter at medical meetings.

Those who now only come as a listener or networker are potential future presenters and can, with this book, also start to learn how to get ready for that moment that you are asked to be on stage.

This book will be your guide and aid to make your future medical meetings even more successful.

Amsterdam, The Netherlands   Jim A. Reekers
March 2010

Contents

Optimal Communication Circumstances

1

Contents

Oral communication is the most powerful way to deliver a message or to present information. The ability to offer important medical content is something, but to give life to that content demands an effective oral presentation. Oral communication is the substance of medical meetings. In the following chapters, you will learn how to improve your presentation skills, but there is much more that goes into making a presentation successful.

There are three parts involved in oral communication:

- **The transmitter**: you
- **The medium**: the environment
- **The receiver**: the audience

The transmitter is, of course, the most important part, without which there is no communication. However, the other two elements also have their valuable roles to play and are discussed in this chapter.

1.1
The Medium

1.1.1
Visual Aids

Visual aids are a significant component of many oral presentations. This includes the use of chalkboards, dry-erase boards, flip charts, slide projectors, overhead projectors

J.A. Reekers, *Presenting at Medical Meetings*,
DOI: 10.1007/978-3-642-12408-2_1, © Springer-Verlag Berlin Heidelberg 2010

and computer programmes. They should always be meaningful, creative and interesting to help the speaker communicate the message. Visual aids should also be adapted to the size of the audience. For presentations at medical meetings, PowerPoint slides are used in almost all instances, which means that the beamer and computer should be high quality. A beamer will decline in quality over time due to ageing of the lamp; therefore, regular maintenance is essential. A beamer is best positioned on the ceiling rather than a table to avoid obstruction of the projection on the screen by the presenter or a latecomer. Furthermore, some older beamers with loud ventilators may distract from your presentation. Of course, there is not much that can be done about an unpredictable beamer once on site, but giving your feedback to the organisers may help them with future presentations.

The computer from which you present is also important. It is well known that not all versions of PowerPoint are compatible with each other. This is particularly true with older vs. newer versions; a newer version might alter the display of your original presentation and result in either unrecognisable or even missing slides. Therefore, it is best to prepare your presentation in one of the recent PowerPoint versions and, of course, always perform a trial run beforehand, either in the preview room or on the actual computer in the presentation room.

Playing movies during your presentation may raise further issues. As described in Sect. 3.10 of Chap. 3, you should be strict with your use of movies; however, there are occasions when they can support the communication of a complicated message. To play a movie, the computer should have media software, which is available in numerous formats and versions. If you do not try the movie ahead of time and your movie has an incompatible extension, you can easily run into problems. It is often difficult, and sometimes impossible, to convert your movie to a different format just before your presentation. In theory, the organisers should always ensure that the most common media software programmes are available on their computers as well as the software to convert movie formats, if necessary. This, however, is almost never the case. It can be quite frustrating to face a computer expert on site who adamantly informs you that your chosen format does not comply with the available (sometimes limited) software. Organisers have selected what, in their expert opinion, is best and should therefore be used by you. However, they can fail to inform you of this beforehand.

It is best to contact the meeting organisers ahead of the meeting for details on their presentation software (PowerPoint, media programmes, etc.). If this approach does not produce a satisfactory outcome (as is the case in my experience), I would urge you to let them know; your feedback could bring about a positive change. Perhaps they can make such information available, either on their Web site or in correspondence, well in advance of the meeting; another solution may be to set international standards for computer presentations.

The organisers of the meeting are responsible for creating an optimal environment for you to perform, and you should not have to be confronted with such issues shortly before holding your presentation. This small service can prove a great help to all involved.

Then, of course, there is the Apple, a great computer with superb visual and graphic design capabilities but a disaster at most meetings. The standard system at 99% of medical meetings is the personal computer (IBM-style PC) and your Apple presentation will just not work – even if they say that it will. Do not take that risk. I have seen several Apple presentations freeze and crash, destroying a talk completely.

Regarding the use of your personal laptop computer for the on site presentation, this is generally no longer allowed at larger meetings as connecting and disconnecting them takes too much time and interrupts the flow of a session. Nevertheless, this is sometimes still permitted at smaller, more informal meetings. Most of the time, however, an internal local-area network (LAN) system requires you simply to bring your presentation to a central point, the preview room, as discussed in Sect. 3.14 of Chap. 3.

1.1.2
Audio

When speaking to an audience of more than 30–40 people, you will need a microphone. The following alternatives are available:

- *Microphone on the lectern.* This is a static system and requires the distance between the speaker and the microphone to be maintained for even sound quality. For instance, when turning your head to look at your slides, the sound might be lost and when standing too close to the microphone, the sound might become too loud.
- *Microphone on the lapel.* This option gives you more freedom to move and turn your head. However, the sound quality and volume can be erratic.
- *Microphone with behind-the-ear headset.* This looks modern and offers the best sound quality. It allows you the freedom to walk around and move away from the lectern. This provides an ideal solution at special occasions, as discussed in the section on blending speech and visual content of Chap. 5.
- *Handheld microphone.* An advantage of this method is that the speaker can be clearly identified, for instance, in panel discussions. However, this is rather old fashioned and static.

1.1.3
Accessories

- *Water.* It is always good to have a glass of still water nearby to ease a dry throat. In this case, it is best to avoid sparkling water as well as milk; these will not help your voice.
- *Pointer.* A pointer with a bright red or green dot is important for highlighting items in your presentation. Should the provided pointer have a weak dot, ask for a replacement. Using the onscreen mouse pointer is discouraged as an accidental click will display the next slide. Returning to a previous slide can, on most lecterns, prove to be a drama.

1.1.4
The Lecture Room

This might seem a triviality, but the significance of the lecture room should not be underestimated. As is the case with the presentation software, you obviously have no influence on this, but it is still part of your presentation. Ideally, the lecture room should adequately accommodate your audience. At larger meetings, however, you sometimes simply have to make do with what is available. I once found myself holding a small technical workshop for 20 people in a 600-seat auditorium. This was a lost cause. Ask the organisers about the size of the room and clearly communicate your needs.

A room that is too small will also prove counterproductive. Having the participants spill out into the corridors and blocking entrances is a disturbance to all involved. Some will leave early if there is no space or, worse still, if the air conditioning is not efficient enough for the large group. Sometimes this is inevitable, but organisers should try to better judge the room allocation by considering the importance of the topic or speaker. You could, of course, tell the organisers that a larger room may be required because you expect a high turnout for your lecture. On the other hand, you could be perceived as pompous, especially if you are wrong, so approach with caution.

Reinforcing speech levels and controlling noise and reverberation are the ultimate acoustical goals of lecture room design to achieve high speech intelligibility. Again, this is out of your control, but when attending a meeting at a purpose-built centre, this is almost always fine. That said, there are situations that you should be made aware of to allow for appropriate planning. Lecturing at a dinner needs special preparation and should only be held by experienced and charismatic speakers to keep the audience's attention. The same is true for lecturing in loud environments or spaces with untraditional seating, like a public place.

- Generally, the size of the lecture room should match the character, content and ambition of the lecture.

1.2
The Receiver

The receiver is your audience. There could be many reasons why you are giving this particular lecture. So, first and foremost, be sure to talk about the right topic to the right audience. Although this seems obvious, it is not always given proper consideration. If you give a medical lecture on molecular imaging to an audience of general physicians just because the meeting organiser is your best friend or has a personal interest in the topic, this will satisfy neither you nor your audience. Always try to ascertain the interests of your audience as well as their level of medical knowledge. You can subsequently adjust your presentation for a better chance of success.

Some other items for your particular attention are as follows:

- Do not make your audience sit in complete darkness when you hold a presentation; you will almost certainly lose all contact. Currently, PowerPoint slides can be viewed in a well-lit room.
- Let the audience know that you are aware of who they are if you do not belong to the same medical group or background.
- Make a reference to a person or organisation related to both yourself and your audience.
- Never act cleverer than your audience. Needless to say, you are the expert, but you will lose part of your audience if you linger on this point. Being arrogant and patronising is the biggest mistake to make.

This is a true story that was told to me first hand. A well-known vascular surgeon was invited to give a speech in Korea. As is often the case with experienced and renowned speakers, he completely relied on his years of experience to pull him through. He planned to arrive just a few hours before his lecture and depart the next morning. He boarded the plane and landed at the airport with a few hours delay, where a nervous Korean representative from the meeting organisation was already waiting for him, holding a sign with the organisation's name on it. He was driven directly to the meeting place, where he handed in his PowerPoint and was guided on stage to give his presentation – the only presentation in English in the session. He did not see anybody he knew from previous meetings, which surprised him only in hindsight, his long intercontinental flight dulling his curiosity. He gave his lecture on a vascular surgery topic and was met with a polite applause. There were no questions, so he left to his hotel. After a few hours, one of his old Korean contacts phoned him at the hotel to ask where he was as he had a lecture to give. It turned out that he had just held a specialised medical lecture to an audience of airplane engineers – both meetings hosted by the same organisers.

The following are a few more points:

- For smaller audiences or for special lectures, it is advisable to be present in the room as the participants arrive. Greeting them or initiating conversation with a few individuals will create a more relaxed atmosphere.
- Be punctual; nothing is more annoying than a speaker who arrives or starts late.

Finish on time; it is extremely difficult (and rare) to keep the full attention of the audience for an extended length of time.

Planning Your Presentation

2

Contents

There are many types of presentations at medical meetings, each with their individual ground rules. With scientific presentations, a speaker is given a specific time slot in a session. Scientific presenters submit their papers on their own initiative and are then usually selected by peer review and are self-funded. For most of the other lectures discussed in this chapter, the speakers are almost always invited based on their reputation in the field.

2.1
Why Me?

It will help a lot with your preparation if you understand clearly why, of all potential speakers, you are invited. It will determine your starting point for preparation, and it will direct the tune of your lecture. Of course, you can just think that every meeting needs some "great" names in its faculty to make the event more interesting for

J.A. Reekers, *Presenting at Medical Meetings*,
DOI: 10.1007/978-3-642-12408-2_2, © Springer-Verlag Berlin Heidelberg 2010

participants. However, I think that this top-down approach is not the best starting point for preparing a lecture.

Routine can make you lazy. I have learned over the years that great names are not always synonymous with great speakers and vice versa. Often, established and famous speakers at medical meetings place too much trust in their experience and are seen to repeat old lectures, with minor changes, for years.

Generally, speakers in the circuit who speak at more than eight different medical meetings annually cannot be original at each of them. Of course, this is not true of all famous speakers.

For the organisers of medical meetings, it is often difficult to bypass these "dinosaurs" as they bring with them a cloud of distinction that can add to the prestige of the meeting. A "preliminary", sometimes called "invited", faculty is often a teaser in the first announcement of a meeting. It is not unusual for the final faculty to be much smaller, lacking the important names from the first announcement. Is this cheating? Actually, it is, but it happens.

Sometimes a speaker is "hot" because the speaker has just written a breakthrough paper or has published an important book. Often, however, it is not clear why other speakers are seen as hot or indispensable to the meeting.

A really bad habit of a number of meetings is selling slots within their official programme to the industry partners to present the latest, or sometimes last year's, "scientific" news about their products or devices, and you are asked to be the industry spokesperson or, as discussed in Sect. 7.2 of Chap. 7, the frontman. This is misleading as the participants of the meeting are not made aware of industry participation. These company-sponsored presentations should be separate from the main programme in clearly identifiable satellite symposia under the auspices of an independent programme committee. Moreover, the name of the sponsoring company should clearly appear next to the presentation, and you as a speaker should be aware of what you are and are not going to present.

So, be absolutely clear why you are invited before you start with your preparation.

2.2
Some Basic Rules for Preparation

If you have determined why you are invited, always ask yourself two basic questions before you start preparing a presentation:

- For which audience am I doing this?
- How should I do this?

2.2.1
For Which Audience Am I Doing This?

First determine the purpose and goals of the meeting. An educational meeting is different from a scientific meeting. The structure and style of your lecture will also depend on this. Know your audience to avoid giving a lecture about barbequing to a group of vegetarians.

So always keep in mind who has invited you, why they invited you and what they expect from you. What is the knowledge and skill level of the audience? And more importantly, what is their level of English or any other language you are presenting in.

If your audience is expected to have a basic level of the English language, prepare your talk and slides in basic English.

Avoid difficult words and abbreviations, something that should in fact apply to every presentation.

What I always find very useful is just asking the organiser, which is usually also the person who invites you, what he/she expects from you. What kind of presentation they had in mind. Try to find out about the content they expect you to cover. Make some notes and confirm what you have discussed by e-mail, so there will be no surprises.

Maybe they have seen one of your previous lectures and they are now looking for a copy–paste lecture. Always worn them that none of your lectures are identical and that you will always update any lecture you give, even if you don't. By this you temper to high expectations. They should know that you are more than a one lecture person.

2.2.2
The Lecture Format

There are several ways you can construct your lecture. For a scientific lecture, the format is fixed; you have hardly any option to play with your creativity.

For other kind of lectures, there are several formats to organise and plan your lecture. Try to find a format that will be best for your lecture.

Chronological format. Your lecture follows a timeline. This is a good way to give an overview of a certain treatment, to show how one step comes after the other and to end at what the current state of the art is. You can then extend the timeline to the future. Chronologically, the lecture follows what was, what is and what will come.

This format is mandatory if your lecture is a summary of a medical career, like in a laudation. Also, this format can be useful for including new ideas.

Problem format. Your lecture is organised around a medical problem. In this format, you can bring or suggest solutions related to these problems. This format can be used for many occasions and is especially useful if you want to stimulate discussion.

Technology format. Your lecture is organised around a technical solution or innovation. This format is good for practical educational lectures or workshops or "how-to-do" lectures.

Case study format. Your lecture is organised around a few patient histories. This format is appropriate for teaching clinical knowledge but has less impact for a larger audience.

Knowledge format. Your lecture is organised to summarise the latest science. This format should be used for a state-of-the-art lecture. Remember that to engage everybody and to have the maximum impact, the format should be easy to follow, easy to digest and easy to remember. It is not about your knowledge but what you are able to communicate.

Argument format. Your lecture is organised around pros and cons. This format can be used to illustrate an ongoing debate or scientific discussion. This format should or can have an open ending.

Rhetorical format. Your lecture is organised around questions and answers. In this format, you ask the questions that are likely to be foremost in the minds of your audience, and then you answer these questions. This is again a great teaching tool, but you have to be a real expert on the topic to master this.

Of course, you can play around with these formats to find your own style, but if you are just starting as a lecturer I would advise you to stay close to one of these formats.

2.2.3
Starting a Lecture

Start to think of a title that will arouse curiosity. Most of the time, the title of your presentation will cover your scientific work, like "Midterm Results from the Barit Study". There is just not much you can do about this. A title like "Everything You Always Wanted to Know About the Midterm Results of the Barit Study" is not appropriate and also not appreciated by a scientific audience.

If you are an invited speaker, look carefully at the given title and make suggestions to change it to something that sounds more appealing if necessary. However, do not make it too flashy; this will only create expectations of a glitz-and-glamour show.

- For instance, changing a title like *"How to Teach Anatomy to a Third-Grade Medical Student"* to *"Beyond Textbook Anatomy for Third-Grade Medical Students"* or *"A New World in Third-Grade Medical Anatomy"* will make it sound more interesting.

However, *"The Dazzling World of Third-Grade Medical Anatomy"* is a bit over the top.

During preparation always keep in mind the universal speaker's law.

The Universal Speaker's Law

Tell them what you are going to tell them.
Tell them.
Tell them what you told them.

- Tell them what you are going to tell them: *Outline of your presentation.*
- Tell them: *Your material and data in detail.*
- Tell them what you told them: *Summarise your material and data and finish your presentation.*

For every lecture, it is important to emphasise the crucial points using different illustrations to drive those points home. If you want an audience to remember the essential points of your lecture, you have to make each point in three to six different ways.

All experienced lecturers do this. Just look for it when you hear a great speaker.

From ancient Greece to the late nineteenth century rhetoric was a central part of Western education, filling the need to train public speakers and writers to move audiences to action with arguments.

There are five canons of rhetoric: *memory, invention, delivery, style and arrangement*; they all should be part of your preparation and your final lecture. In general, they should all be used to create the right composition as a means for moving audiences.

During your preparation for a presentation, you are mainly organising the arguments.

2.3
Preparing Your Presentation

2.3.1
Scientific Presentations

Speakers in a scientific session are selected through peer review. A session is organised around a mutual theme and is intended to encourage the exchange of new scientific knowledge, to create a podium for research groups and to stimulate scientific discussion. The aim in a scientific session is to get your message across to other professionals and to discuss your results.

If there are six speakers in a 1-h scientific session, which is quite usual, in theory everybody has 10 min gross presenting time. Walking on and off stage, including the chairperson's introduction, is about 1 min. One ore two questions after your talk will take about 1–2 min. So, a 10-min scientific slot is actually only 7–8 min of net presentation time.

At most quality meetings, the chairs are required to be strict, especially in terms of timekeeping; sessions often follow one another in quick succession, and punctuality is of great importance. Also the industry sponsored satellite symposia, as seen at larger medical meetings, should start on time as this industry participation is essential for the finances of almost every larger meeting.

For a scientific presentation, the structure, next to the data, is the most important issue. It is a delicate balance between what to tell and what not to tell, that is, which information carries the message and which will confuse or distract.

I would advise you to start with the results and conclusions and work backward to the introduction. The results, especially the conclusions, are what you want to communicate.

There are a few indispensable slides in any scientific presentation.

Basic slides for a scientific presentation	Description
Research questions	Rationale for doing this study
Study design	Retrospective, randomised, and so on
Inclusion and exclusion criteria	Describe the study population
Materials and method	Describe patients, technique, statistics, and so on
Results	Based on good statistics
Conclusions	In relation to the research questions

In theory six slides will do.

Add:

- One slide to introduce yourself and your co-workers
- One slide to disclose any conflicts of interest from yourself, your group or institute

And you are done.

- Maybe add one slide to expand the materials and method
- One slide extra for results, if you really need that

So, a basic scientific presentation is no more than eight slides.

- Two slides for tables, figures or graphics

If you also need to show tables, figures or graphics,
A scientific presentation has a maximum of 12 slides.

2.3.2
Invited Lectures

Being invited for a lecture is a great honour, and one should try as much as possible to live up to the expectations of the inviting organization. Try to understand what is expected of you. Is this an educational lecture, a state-of-the-art lecture or an honorary lecture? Are you the only speaker in the session? If there are other speakers, what are their topics? How is the session structured? Find out how much time is allocated to each speaker and if there is room for discussion.

It is surprising to see how many speakers accept an invitation without even asking the most basic questions that will determine how one is going to prepare the invited lecture.

> ### Checklist for Invited Speakers
>
> - Location of the meeting
> - Dates of the meeting and the lecture
> - Audience
> - Type of lecture
> - Topic of the lecture
> - Allocated speaker time
> - Session structure
> - Who the other speakers are
> - Topics of the other speakers

If there is a chance that the speakers in a session have overlapping topics or areas, contact them in advance to discuss the exact content of their presentations. There is nothing more embarrassing than hearing the speaker who precedes you present parts, sometimes major parts, of the talk you are about to give, sometimes even with different conclusions.

This should be avoided at all costs, so contact the other speakers in your session to avoid this eventuality.

Like every performance, the outcome very much depends on the preparation. The few who are talented enough to improvise and get away with such a situation have actually missed out on a career as a politician. Most of us are just physicians without such talents.

Invited lectures can have many purposes and should be prepared accordingly. There are educational lectures, state-of-the-art lectures, personal lectures and keynote lectures. I think most invitations can be placed under one of these types. Choose a lecture format that will fit with the purpose and content of your lecture (Sect. 2.1.2). The other important thing to know, right from the start, is how much speaking time you have and at what time in the programme the lecture is planned.

2.3.3
Education Lecture or a State-of-the-Art Lecture

For an education lecture or a state-of-the-art lecture, 20 min are optimal. These lectures should contain no anecdotes, no emotions and no personal commitment with the audience. Anyhow, if you are not able to condense an educational message in 20 min, you will lose your audience.

You work from start to finish in a regular flat tempo. Your lecture should always contain information on the most recent and up-to-date medical science. Referring to publications older than 10 years can only be allowed when you compare historical data with recent publications. For these kind of lectures, always make a list of points you want the audience to take home. It is a good habit to end with one slide called "Take-Home points" that summarises the bullet points you want your audience to remember.

2.3.4
Keynote and Personal Lectures

Keynote and personal lectures, on the other hand, should contain anecdotes, emotions and personal commitment with the audience. From start to finish, these lectures should contain rhythm, be upbeat, pull the rope and let it go, and provide highlights and quiet moments.

A big crescendo at the end will make your lecture an event an audience will remember for a long time. I know this from personal experience.

If people still remember "that" lecture after years, probably having forgotten about the exact content completely, you still have achieved your goal.

A keynote or personal lecture is very much all about you. Of course, the content must be high class but what remains is the moment.

Never repeat a keynote or personal lecture at another meeting because after one performance you will find that the soul is out of your lecture, and that it does not rock and roll anymore.

Why this is, I have no idea.

2.4
Lecture Timing

So, now that you have determined the kind of lecture you are going to give, you should start to plan your lecture time accordingly.

Although already discussed, I must reiterate one basic rule: For every presentation at a medical congress, a specific time slot is allocated. An open time slot for a presentation is extremely rare.

Staying within your time slot not only is polite but also is essential so you do not cause yourself and the following presenters serious inconvenience. Nevertheless, going overtime is the most often encountered problem at any meeting but actually the easiest to overcome.

Just buy a watch with large numbers and hands and place it on the lectern so that you can see how much time is left. Alternatively, rehearse your lecture a few times at home with an egg timer.

Remember, on the other hand, that an undertimed lecture is always embarrassing, especially when you are an invited speaker.

A rule of thumb is that

- A 10-min scientific lecture should use a maximum of 12 slides.
- A 20-min educational lecture uses between 20 and 30 slides.
- A 30-min personal or keynote lecture uses a maximum of 60 slides.

For a scientific 10-min lecture slot, there is 7–8 min presentation time and 2 min question-and-answer period.

It is unsatisfying to present scientific study data you have been working on for a long time, about which you are enthusiastic, and not being able to discuss it with an interested scientific audience. The question-and-answer section will again give you the opportunity to highlight the most important points.

2.5
Humour

2.5.1
A Scientific Presentation is not the Right Medium for Jokes

This is perhaps the right time and place to say a few words about humour. You should think about this when you start to plan your presentation. Humour can sometimes be effective during an invited lecture; it can arouse attention, can wake up the audience and can be a nice bridge to the next item in your talk. However, keep in mind that pre-prepared humour, especially jokes, often work counterproductively and distract from your message. Would you like to be remembered for your jokes or for the content and message of your lecture? I would advise that you only start with humour when you really feel free on stage and even then … be careful.

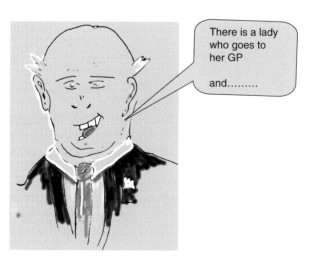

There was once a famous chest radiologist who was also an excellent speaker and lecturer. Furthermore, he was the author of some famous textbooks. I only saw him speak once, a long time ago, when I was still a junior. Although I had already planned to go to his lecture, I was repeatedly told by many not to miss it. Next to being a great speaker, he was also known as a notorious narrator of dirty jokes during his lectures. The format was the same every time: one borderline joke in the middle of the lecture and one over-the-line joke at the end of the lecture, so everybody stayed until the end. The hall was full, and the lecturer did not disappoint his fans. To this day, I still remember both jokes vividly, but I have not the slightest clue what his lecture was about. As I told you, he gave great lectures, but his audience only came for the jokes – a waste of time and energy and a missed career as an entertainer.

However, it is the latest craze in the name of humour that is the most distracting and unprofessional: to dot your presentation with "funny" clips from YouTube. This is simply out of harmony with the purpose of being on stage in a scientific function.

Although some of the movies can be amusing, show them on another occasion.

Stop doing this; you are *not* funny.

You are not the medical joker, or is that your ambition in life? Humour and science just do not mix well.

2.6
Planning Your Visual Performance

2.6.1
How to Dress

For every medical meeting, there is a dress code. Only a few can legally escape this – those in a special category, which hardly anybody reaches.

I once attended a lecture by a famous thoracic surgeon who had operated on the rich and famous. When he came on stage in a T-shirt, jeans, sneakers and a baseball cap, many thought that he was the room assistant checking the microphone. It was only when he started talking that people recognised him.

I will not provide you with individual dress codes for every medical specialty in the world as this also changes over time and is very much dependent on the local colours. A T-shirt, jeans, sneakers and a baseball cap, however, are not appropriate attire anywhere in the world of medical meetings, often not even after hours.

Men: Men cannot go wrong with a dark-coloured suit and a clean shirt. Do not go for fashionable tailor-made suits unless you are Italian. They are the only doctors who know how to wear and present themselves in such a suit in a natural way. This is something you cannot learn if you were not born there. Most of us will look like a peacock.

Your tie should not be funny, brightly coloured or oversize.

Do not wear so-called power ties. Nothing in your attire should detract from your message. Shoes, although most of the time under the lectern, should match; again, sneakers should not be worn, a crime I have witnessed many times in the United States. Socks should not be white; this is especially annoying if you are sitting on the bench of a forum discussion.

Men are free to choose their own underwear.

Women: Women are less bound by conventions than men. The main message is

> **Do not wear anything which might detract from the main reason of you being on stage.**

I will not go into detail here, but I think the message is clear enough. This is also true for jewellery and other accessories. Do not bring your Prada handbag with you on stage (even more important when you are a man).

And, once again, before I forget, women are also free to choose their own underwear.

2.7
Make Your Own Audience

If you are a speaker in a scientific session, it is sometimes a good idea to ask some of your colleagues to come along. If there are no questions from the audience, they can conjure up one or two pre-prepared questions to give you and your talk maximum exposure.

Finally

Prepare your talk in advance; it needs time to condense, to sink in. When you look back on your proposed presentation after 2 weeks, you will almost always recognise things that should be changed. It is often obvious if a presentation had been prepared the day before; it simply looks careless, with missing words and spelling mistakes. Often, this goes hand in hand with an equally careless speaker performance.

One month is the minimum preparation time for a good presentation.

For tips on how to prepare the perfect PowerPoint presentation and how to become an excellent speaker, please go to the next chapters.

Summary

Always ask the three basic questions:

- — Why me?
- — For which audience am I doing this?
- — How should I do this?

- Never forget the universal speaker's law.
- Find out all about your session before you start.
- Plan your lecture time.
- Be careful with humour.
- Follow the dress code of the meeting.
- One month is the minimal preparation time for a good presentation.

How to Make a Perfect PowerPoint Presentation

3

Contents

I have seen countless badly organised medical meeting slide presentations in which the message got completely lost. Those of you who have visited a medical meeting before know that an important aspect of any scientific presentation is showing slides. In the old days, slides were expensive, labour intensive and fragile, not to

J.A. Reekers, *Presenting at Medical Meetings*,
DOI: 10.1007/978-3-642-12408-2_3, © Springer-Verlag Berlin Heidelberg 2010

mention the pure weight of glass-mounted slides, which limited the number that could be carried to a meeting. The last was not so bad actually as it was also a practical limitation to the number of slides one could bring to show. It forced the presenter to make a preselection of slides at home. Including too many slides in a presentation is a problem discussed in this chapter.

In past years, slides were always made by either your secretary or a medical illustrator and were produced by the hospital audiovisual service and used over and over again to save money. Slides had to be ordered weeks in advance. A slide was not a "ready-made disposable", but something you had to think about because you had to use it time and time again. Even projecting the slides was a challenge as they had to be turned around and placed upside down in the projector carrousel for them to be seen the right way.

As the slides constituted a large and heavy volume, many doctors did not carry them in their hand luggage. However, glass-mounted slides that had been in the freight compartment of an airplane often showed some condensation, which was then heated by the projector lamp during a presentation. This produced the most fantastic psychedelic effects as the condensation started to move around between the glass plates.

Glass mounting was an absolute necessity because the strong projectors used in larger auditoria in those days simply burned any unmounted slide if the speaker remained on one slide longer than 30 s. Although the old slides had many disadvantages, the main advantage was that one really had to think about what to present. Also, the graphics and today's audiovisual possibilities were non-existent, which I sometimes think was not such a bad thing.

Currently, anything is possible; anyone can be a graphic designer or, even worse, an artist. This is often not an advantage as in many slide presentations the message is completely overwhelmed by words flying in and out, conclusions crawling in, multicoloured artwork and funny clips. Sometimes, it is a competition to see who can get as much information as possible on one slide. Usually, a slide like this is introduced by the presenter as "on this slightly crowded slide, you can clearly see … ". Well, usually you cannot see anything at all.

There are clear annual trends, such as a blue background with white text, a green background with brown text, clouds, various fonts, illegible fonts and many more. I have seen it all. The biggest mistake is to forget that PowerPoint is a tool designed to support your presentation, not to *be* your presentation. You are the presenter. You are the focus, not your slides. You have the leading role, and you need to retain that role. No "coloured light show" can mask a weak presentation. If you do not do your job, PowerPoint cannot save you. It only makes a bad presentation worse.

I once walked with a friend to a buffet counter at a meeting, where we encountered one of the old congress veterans. We had both known him for years. He was accompanied by a much younger, good-looking lady. We had a short chat, after which we continued our walk. "Is that his new wife?" I asked, "Yes", my friend replied. "New wife, but still the same old slides".

3.1
Basic Rules

The following are ten basic rules of how to make the perfect slide presentation for any medical lecture:

1. Never follow a trend but create one and stick to your own style.
2. Each slide has to carry a message that supports or adds to your oral presentation.
3. A slide is not an autocue. If you are only going to read from the slides, you might as well just send them, ask the chair to read them and stay home.
4. Your oral presentation, not your PowerPoint slides, is the carrier of the core message.
5. Do not use the media to hide yourself. The audience came to *see* you.
6. A slide must not distract people from your performance.
7. Limit the number of slides to no more than 10–12 for a 10-min presentation.
8. Limit the number of words on each slide; six to eight is usually ideal.
9. A PowerPoint should *enhance* your presentation not *be* your presentation.
10. Less is more.

3.2
Fonts

If people cannot read your slides from the back of the room, the font is too small. If people are squinting during your presentation to try to make out what is on the slide, you have lost your audience. In my experience, you must use at least a 30-point font.

Use appropriate fonts. I recommend the following:

- A sans serif font for titles (e.g. Arial, Verdana, Helvetica, Tahoma, etc.)
- A serif font for bullets or body text (e.g. Times New Roman, Garamond, Goudy, Palatino, etc.)
- A sans serif font customarily for chart tables

The serifs help you recognise the characters (and thus the words) faster. It makes the text more readable.

Use a template with a standardised font throughout the whole presentation.

Slides might look fancy or artistic when you use a "romantic" font, but you will lose the attention of your audience because your slides do not communicate well. The text must be obvious and easy to read. Remember that you are not there to present your artistic alter ego; your task is to communicate a message.

We are all trained in automatic reading, which means that even at a glance you recognise a word in its correct context. However, if your audience is concentrating on reading your presentation rather than absorbing it, they will need much more time to understand the sentence or context, and you will have lost them.

How to do it

> ## The conclusions of the Barit study
>
> - Drinking milk does not prevent fractures
> - Cow milk is better than sheep milk
> - Calcium and Plaster are age dependent

Title: Verdana, 32 point
Bullets: Times New Roman, 32 point

How not to do it

> ## *The conclusions of the Barit study*
>
> - *Drinking milk does not prevent fractures*
> - *Cow milk is better than sheep milk*
> - *Calcium and Plaster are age dependent*

Title: Arial Black, 32 point, Italic and Shadow
Bullets: Arial Black, 24 point, Italic and Shadow

How to make it difficult for the audience

> ## *The conclusions of the Barit study*
>
> - *Drinking milk does not prevent fractures*
> - *Cow milk is better than sheep milk*
> - *Calcium and Plaster are age dependent*

Title: Comic Sans MS, 36 point, Italic and Shadow
Bullets: Comic Sans MS, 32 point, Italic and Shadow

Unreadable

> *The conclusions of the Barit study*
>
> * *Drinking milk does not prevent fractures*
> * *Cow milk is better than sheep milk*
> * *Calcium and Plaster are age dependent*

3.2.1 Font Size

The larger the font size is, the better it is. Remember, your slides must be legible, even from the back of the room.

Obviously, it depends on the size of the room, the size of the screen, and so on. This is precisely why you cannot afford to leave this to chance. You must test your slides and make certain that they are readable. The more words you use, the smaller the font will be and the less legible the words will be.

For example, if you use Verdana:

- Title Verdana, 40 point.
- A good subtitle or bullet point size should be Verdana, 32 point.
- Content text should be no smaller than Verdana, 24 point.

Combining small font sizes with bold or italics is not recommended.

Do not sacrifice readability for style.

Do Not Capitalise Everything.

It only

- Makes text hard to read
- Conceals acronyms
  - Disallows the use of uppercasing for Emphasis

> THE CONCLUSIONS OF THE BARIT STUDY
>
> * DRINKING MILK DOES NOT PREVENT FRACTURES
> * COW MILK IS BETTER THAN SHEEP MILK
> * CALCIUM AND PLASTER ARE AGE DEPENDENT

Avoid capitalisation unless it is a title. Sentence capitalisation is much easier to read. This is especially valid when dealing with many bullet points.

Italics

- Used for "quotes"
- Used to highlight thoughts or ideas
- Used for book, journal or magazine titles

3.3
Visual Content

Avoid paragraphs or long blocks of text. If you really must use a paragraph, then whittle it down to the bare essentials. Use an excerpt – a couple of sentences. Emphasise the important words. Put the text block by itself on a single slide.

How not to Do it

> The Barit study was a multi-centre study to investigate the use of milk in prevention of fractures in octogenarians. The study was sponsored by the national institute of natural farming, the NINF, and was initiated by 2 individuals. The primary investigator was C. Milk MD at the institute for global agriculture. A total of 2,000 octogenarians participated in this study.

Too much text looks busy and is hard to read. Why read it when you are going to be told what it says? Our reading speed does not match our listening speed; hence, the audience ends up confused.

There are a few ways to improve this slide.

If you think it is absolutely vital to have a whole text block because it is a quotation or a well-known or historic text, like the Declaration of Independence, and you cannot change the order of the text, you can use serif or highlighting with bold or colour.

Keep the original Layout

> The **Barit study** was a multi-centre study to investigate the <u>use of milk in prevention of fractures</u> in octogenarians. The study was sponsored by the national institute of natural farming, the NINF, and was initiated by 2 individuals. The primary investigator was C Milk MD at the institute for global agriculture. A total of <u>2,000 octogenarians</u> participated in this study.

or better

> # The Barit study
>
> - Multi- center study in 2000 octogenarians
> - Use of milk in prevention of fractures in octogenarians
> - Primary investigator: C. Milk, MD, institute for global agriculture.
>
> Sponsor: **national institute of natural farming, NINF.**

Now you have the same information but it is *easily readable!*

<u>Avoid detailed reports in your presentation</u>

It is all about communication and readability. The most recent trend is using fancy mobile phone text or Twitter language in PowerPoint slides. Your audience over a certain age will not understand what you mean. It just looks ugly and distracts from the message. So, do not follow this trend.

Clinical outcome for all patients at 4-year follow-up

Is now sometimes written as

Clinical outcome 4 all ptt @ 4 years FU

3.4
Pointless Motion

One of the main disadvantages of PowerPoint is the really endless animation options. You can be anything from a graphic designer to an animation director. If people come up to you after your lecture with questions about how you were able to create certain animations in your slides and are not interested in the content of your lecture, you have just killed your lecture with pointless motion.

Avoid fancy slide transitions and fly-ins; they get old quickly, and they distract from the real reason you are there. I strongly recommend that you keep things simple. A basic dissolve from one slide to another is sufficient. Have all your bullets appear at once rather than one at a time or, even worse, word by word.

Avoid sound effects; they serve no other purpose than annoying the audience and distracting from your presentation.

Cut down the number of slides. You do not need a transcript of your speech with every point and sub-point. People are only going to remember the major points anyway.

Avoid white backgrounds as the white screen can be blinding in a dark room. Dark slides with light coloured text work best.

3.5
Background

The background can be another source of distraction from your presentation. Prominent, "interesting" or funny backgrounds distract from the message.

Choose your background and use the same one on every slide. Changing the style is distracting.

A mono-colour background like blue is better than a picture background.

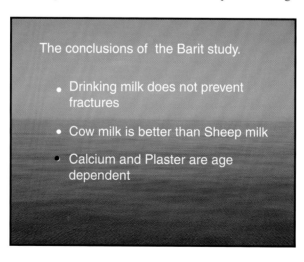

Sometimes, the background makes it difficult to read the text.

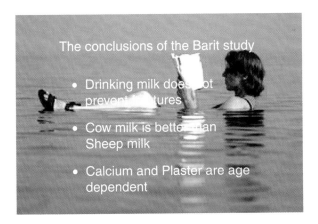

Are you out of your mind?

It is a well-known fact that the most important factor in reading text is …
contrast.

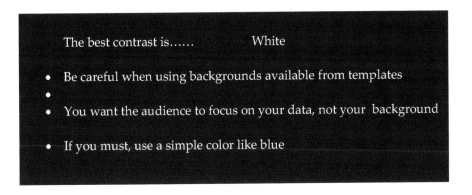

3.6
Colours

Colours in general can be distracting and might have a negative influence on read-ability. Nevertheless, they can also help to create a certain atmosphere. Good general advice is to be careful with colours and not to use too many in one slide. Your slides should not look like an advertisement for a circus.

If you want to combine background colours and text colours, you have to know about the interaction of colours.

Choose high-contrast colours.

A presentation is ineffective if no one can read the text on your slides. Use high-contrasting colours to prevent losing slide text in the background.

For example, white text on a black background has high contrast and is much easier to read than dark blue text on a black background.

However, white on dark background should not be used if the audience is more than 20 ft away. The further away you get, the harder it is to read.

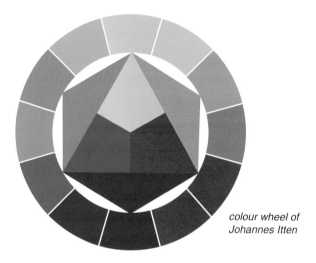

colour wheel of
Johannes Itten

Look at the colour wheel of Johannes Itten for guidance. Colours that are opposite each other on this wheel have the highest contrast. Always match your background with a colour of the highest contrast to improve readability.

This is how the wheel can help you:

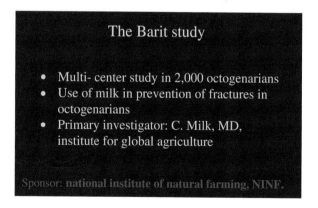

This is a strange colour combination, but it provides good readability. Only the last line (blue) is not a contrasting colour and is therefore unreadable.

It also works vice versa.

The Barit study

- Multi- center study in 2,000 octogenarians
- Use of milk in prevention of fractures in octogenarians
- Primary investigator: C. Milk, MD, institute for global agriculture

Sponsor: **national institute of natural farming, NINF.**

This, however, should never happen.

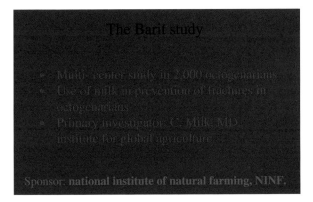

Never use red text or black text on a blue background; it might look okay on your computer screen, but it is horrible on the projector screen.

Finally,

- Reds and oranges are high-energy, but it can be difficult to stay focused on these colours

- Greens, blues, and browns are mellower, but not as attention grabbing

- Reds and greens can be difficult to see for the colour blind

3.7
Graphs and Charts

Graphs and charts are great because they communicate information visually. For this reason, graphs are often used during medical presentations. Graphs or charts can help impress people by getting your point across quickly and visually. However, they can also create a lot of confusion. There are many types of graphs you can use in your presentation. I summarise the most used ones and indicate their use.

3.7.1
Line Graph

Line graphs are used to track changes over short and long periods of time. When smaller changes exist, line graphs are better to use than bar graphs. Line graphs can also be used to compare changes over the same period of time for more than one group.

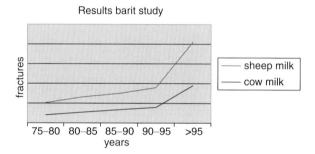

3.7.2
Pie Chart

Pie charts are best to use when you are trying to compare parts of a whole. They do not show changes over time.

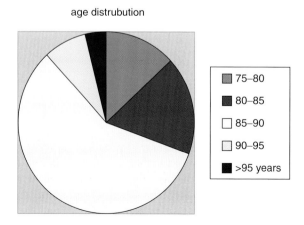

3.7.3
Bar Graph

Bar graphs are used to compare things between different groups or to track changes over time. However, when trying to measure change over time, bar graphs are best when the changes are larger.

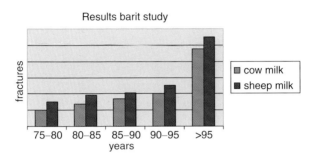

3.7.4
Area Graph

Area graphs are similar to line graphs. They can be used to track changes over time for one or more groups. Area graphs are good to use when you are tracking the changes in two or more related groups that make up one whole category (e.g. age groups).

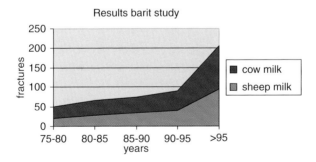

3.7.5
X–Y Plot

X–Y plots are used to determine relationships between the two different things. The *x*-axis is used to measure one event (or variable), and the *y*-axis is used to measure the other. If both variables increase at the same time, they have a positive relationship. If one variable decreases while the other increases, they have a negative relationship. Sometimes, the variables do not follow any pattern and have no relationship.

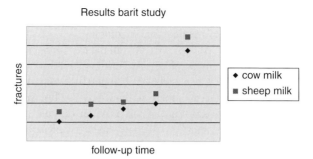

After you have chosen the right graphics make sure that

- The audience can read them.
- The audience understands them immediately.
- They support your presentation.

If you are very much involved in a topic, it might be difficult to see if a graphic presentation is too complicated or needs too much explanation. For graphs and charts, it is important always to pre-test them on somebody who is not familiar with the topic. Just ask a few colleagues if they can understand the slide. And, as with all slides, do not put too much information on one, or your audience will not stay with you.

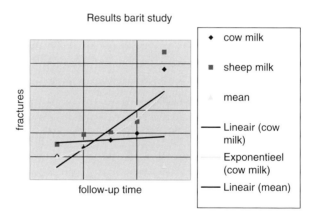

This is much too complicated.

3.8
Illustrations and Pictures

- Use illustrations and pictures only when needed; otherwise, they become distracters instead of communicators.
- They should relate to the message and help make a point.
- Always ask yourself if they make the message clearer.

Limit each slide to one illustration only.

There is a huge variety of medical and medicine-related pictures for download available on the Web. Some of them are free, but the best ones you have to buy. The price depends on the resolution; high-resolution pictures are more expensive. Anything between 5 and 100 € is possible. When you buy them, you also pay for the copyright. Of course, you can use them without paying, but then the picture will show the irremovable prominent logo of the provider on your slide. The cheapest thing you can do is to ask yourself: "Do I really need this picture, and does it add to my presentation?" Most of the time, the answer is negative.

Just google for pictures under *"Funny doctor pics"*, and you will see what I mean.

3.9
Bullet Points

To cover components of an idea

– Keep each bullet to one line, two at the most.
– Limit the number of bullets on a screen to six and only four if there is a large title, logo, picture, and the like. This is known as *cueing.*

You want to *cue* the audience on what you are going to say.

– Cues are a brief *preview.*
– Cues give the audience a *framework* to build on. However, if there is too much text, the audience will not read it.

3.10
Animation

Animation is only applicable to invited speakers and not to presenters of scientific data, who should never use animation.

– Limit animation; too much can be distracting. Be consistent with animation and have all text and photos appear in the same way each time. There are many animation modes, but it is best to use just one throughout. If you do not limit them, the audience will only see the animation and not the message you are trying to get across.

I would also like to say something about the current YouTube pollution, which is simply annoying. People download low-quality YouTube clips and incorporate them into their PowerPoint, almost always with the intention to make their presentation more interesting and lively or just to create the image of being funny.

Most of the time, these clips have no relevance to the topic and are merely there for entertainment. Remember, you are invited to be on stage to communicate a scientific or educational message, not to be the fool of the meeting.

Maybe we should have the opportunity to show these movies to each other during coffee and tea breaks.

Stop showing "funny movies" in powerpoints, please!

3.11
Storyboard

Always use a storyboard to organise your PowerPoint presentation.

I know that there are experienced speakers who prepare their presentation in just 10 min in the preview room, but the result is usually an unstructured lecture. Do not follow their example.

Step 1

If you are an experienced presenter, you can probably skip this first step. Most experienced presenters are already used to making a storyboard in their heads. Nevertheless, it is my experience that if you prepare a storyboard every now and then, it will improve your PowerPoint presentation. Especially if you have the honour of being invited to a prestigious lecture, some reflection on your own performance might be important to get the best out of your presentation.

If you do not have a lot of experience, I would advise you never to start writing a PowerPoint presentation without first making a storyboard outline of what you want to say to your audience. I still think pen and paper are suitable for this, but I admit to being somewhat old fashioned in this matter.

Your storyboard should create a logical flow to your presentation: Tell a story. It must flow easily.

The golden rule of every presentation is to

Tell them what you are going to tell them; tell them; then tell them what you told them.

Start with a good outline.

Think of what you want to accomplish with the presentation. Write down the message you want the audience to remember when they leave the room.

If you are happy with your presentation on the storyboard, let it sit for a couple of days and then look at it again. If you have no idea what it is all about when you pick it up again, you should definitely start again. Normally, you immediately see what you have to change after you pick it up again. Organise and re-organise your presentation until you are satisfied.

3.12
Making Slides

I do not discuss the slide programmes available here. Microsoft PowerPoint is by far the most widely used programme in the world for making presentational slides. I have seen dramatic crashes of other systems, so if you want to use a different one, please check with the local audiovisual support of the meeting. Make sure that it really works before you go on stage.

Instructions about how the PowerPoint programme actually works and should be used are not part of this book. Basic PowerPoint knowledge is, of course, needed and can be learned from many books available on the market. An easy one is PowerPoint for Dummies.

For those who really want to dig deeper into the possibilities of PowerPoint, especially into unexpected graphic and drawing options, I refer to a nice article by Lababede and Meziane called "*Medical Illustration Techniques for PowerPoint*" (American Journal of Roentgenology, April 2007).

The only technical advice I can give you, as I am not really a computer whiz, is always to use the most recently available version of PowerPoint. Using older versions can cause completely incomprehensible slides during projection.

Before I forget, there is something absolutely vital that you have to do when you have finished your PowerPoint, especially as a non-native speaker.

Conclucions

- Drinking milk does not prevend fractures
- Cow milk is beter than sheap milk
- Calcimum and plaster are age dependend

Always use your spell-checker, which is important even when you are a native speaker.

It looks unprofessional to have typing errors in your slides when prevention is just a mouse click away.

3.13
Start with a Presentation

When you start a PowerPoint presentation, the first thing you must do is to target your audience.

If you want to communicate, say, in English, you need to know how experienced your audience is in this language. For a mixed audience, which is often the case at international medical meetings, you should use words understandable to all. Do not use medical slang or rare abbreviations, especially when the majority of the audience is non-native. The basic rule "less is more" is essential for a good presentation.

3.13.1
First Slide

There is an ongoing discussion between the United States and Europe about what the first slide should be. In the United States, it is absolutely mandatory for regulatory Continuing Medical Education (CME) reasons always to start with a disclosure slide of the possible conflicts of interest of the presenter, authors, study group, research department or even the university, along with the presented data or study results. This includes a long list of possible conflicts of interest due to relationships.

Possible relationships

- Employment
- Consultancies
- Honoraria
- Stock
- Grants
- Patents
- Royalties
- Payment

In Europe, this is yet to become mandatory, although I often think it might sometimes clarify some "spectacular" research findings.

So, for a U.S. presentation the declaration of possible interests is always the first slide.

3.13.2
Second Slide

The second slide introduces you, your group, your grant donator if applicable and the title of your presentation. I explained in the previous chapter that a title should be catchy but within certain limits.

The results from the Baritt study

Dr. Highilby Broon, MD

Department of Geriatrics, University of Broondale

On behalf of the Baritt study group

National institute of natural farming

Simply clean and good information

But I also have seen multiple variations on this one.

The spectacular results from the amazing Baritt Study

Dr. Highilby Broon, MD, PhD, FRCP, ESIR, BRIM

University of Broondale

World centre of excellence

You have to convince the audience with your lecture and data, not with your second slide.
The rest of your slides will now follow just naturally.

Just one more tip:

The rule of six

- No more than six lines per slide
- No more than six words per line

One final bit of advice about improving your PowerPoint presentation: Look at how others do it, try to identify their strengths and weaknesses and learn from them. You will see that your PowerPoint will also improve over time. One last item remains to be discussed in this chapter.

3.14
The Preview Room

At many meetings, you are required to send your presentation a few weeks before the meeting starts, which does not allow for any last-minute modifications and changes. I always bring my slides with me to the meeting. Most of the time, they need to have them at least 2 h in advance; do not rush in at the last moment as you will probably find a long queue and only a few available computers.

Be sure to bring a copy of your presentation on a USB flash drive or save a copy on your laptop. Nothing is more embarrassing than having to announce that you have lost your only USB flash drive with the presentation on it.

Go to the preview room and ask the assistant there to help you download your presentation. Ask if this is how it will be shown in the lecture room. If you have movie clips, check that they are compatible with the available system. If they do not run, you have to delete them. I see speakers become annoyed (and much worse) at almost every meeting I attend because of malfunctioning movies. I never use such movies as I do not think that they ever add anything more than a good picture or line drawing. They could perhaps add value to some technical or educational lectures.

After downloading, make sure that your presentation is on the server. It is common that after downloading the presentation the USB flash drive is forgotten in the pre-view room. Be careful; there could be further slides of your presentation saved on it.

The preview room is your final rehearsal without the audience, so take advantage of this and take your time.

Some people think that a preview room is also a social room where you can meet and chat with colleagues and old friends. This should be avoided at all times; it is unpleasant for those who need silence to concentrate and work on their presenta-tions. You might be an experienced lecturer, but many are not.

How to Become a Professional Speaker

4

Contents

J.A. Reekers, *Presenting at Medical Meetings*,
DOI: 10.1007/978-3-642-12408-2_4, © Springer-Verlag Berlin Heidelberg 2010

Some have it, and some don't. Some have a natural way of presenting on stage, while others struggle their way through a presentation. Just accept the fact that not everybody will win an Academy Award for best actor or actress.

While having some natural narrative talent is, of course, helpful, it does not automatically make you an excellent speaker at medical meetings. I have seen gifted people deliver poor presentations. It takes more than some talent; it also takes a great deal of bragging. Even if you are a gifted speaker like Barack Obama, you need to prepare everything in detail and not rely on on-the-spot improvisation. Obama is notorious for his preparation and application of all kinds of electronics – and it pays off.

Can you become an excellent speaker at a medical meeting?

Yes, You Can!!!

It just takes a few basic rules, some training and confidence. Of course, speaking in front of an audience can be terrifying, and for many people it is their number one fear. You can always choose to have a different medical career, simply observing, sitting in the darkness of the lecture room. But, if you want to move upward on the hierarchic ladder of academic medicine, public presentation of your work is a must. If you know the basic rules of presenting, you will see flawed presentations all the time.

Many presentations, according to Bill Wilson, a communication expert, are tornado presentations. They are like real tornadoes; *they are a concentrated gust of wind that sucks.* And like most tornadoes, *they are not planned – they just happen.*

There can be a variety of reasons for giving a presentation at a medical meeting. You could be sent by your department to present results from a scientific trial, or you could be invited by the local organisers or an industry partner to give a specific lecture. Of course, an exotic location could also be a good reason to go or to accept an invitation. The invitation will determine what kind of lecture you will have to give. Nevertheless, sometimes during a presentation I find myself thinking: *Why am I doing this?*

An invitation from a colleague you have known for years can make it difficult to decline. If you really do not want to go, it is always best to say this immediately and not to wait until the final programme is finished. Last-minute cancellations are never appreciated. If for any reason you cannot make it, be honest, and if you are happier with a cooked-up story, be sure to make a note of it.

A colleague of mine was notorious for being on the road all the time. He liked to travel the world, and he was especially interested in remote and exotic places. Because he did not want to miss an opportunity to travel, he accepted all incoming invitations for lectures. It could, however, happen that after acceptance a more attractive invitation arrived. He was then confronted with a double booking in his agenda, so he had to drop the less-interesting travel destination. His tactic was to wait until the last moment and then to contact the organisers of the meeting (he was about to decline) with a cooked-up story. After some years, he had quite a reputation for cancelling at the last moment. Some years ago, he again cancelled a meeting at the last moment with the story that his father had died. He then received a return question asking how many fathers he had because the organisers had already sent their condolences when his father died 2 years ago.

Ok, no more excuses: Let's go for it.

For a good presentation, there is one golden rule:

Prepare — Prepare — Prepare

There are many aspects you have to prepare, but it is the sum of all of them that makes a good lecture. I discuss all of these aspects here one by one.

4.1
The Speaker

The speaker is one of the most important aspects of the presentation. Do not come with a story that you have a weak voice or a monotone voice or whatever. I have seen a presenter who was a genuine stutterer give an excellent presentation despite his handicap. So, give no more excuses.

There are three aspects to consider as a speaker.

Motivation — Credibility — Delivery

4.1.1
Motivation

Motivation is related to the reward you receive for giving a presentation at a medical meeting. If there is no reward, you will lack motivation. A reward might be that your hard work as a research fellow can finally be presented to an audience full of interested colleagues. You feel this and get rewarded. At the other end of the spectrum, the reward could also be that you are again recognised as an eminence and expert in your specific field of medicine. If there is no reward, in other words, if you are sent by a senior or if you are a replacement presenting somebody else's work, you will not have the motivation that is needed for a good speech. It takes a brilliant actor to be convincing without motivation. So, be behind the lectern for the right reasons. Always ask yourself, "Why am I doing this?"

Always try to find a motivation for your upcoming lecture. Also, a nice venue near a sunny beach or being with old friends can be a motivation. Always say, "I am looking forward to my lecture". Never say, "I wish I had never accepted this lecture".

4.1.2
Credibility

Credibility is also important. A speaker and his or her message are accepted by a professional audience only to the degree that the speaker is perceived to be credible.

The speaker's credibility depends on the speaker's trustworthiness, competence and goodwill. A speaker who is well organised, who does not jump back and forth through his or her slides, will usually be considered competent. The speaker who is attractive and dynamic will be seen as more credible than one who is not. The most fundamental factor speakers project is their opinion of themselves. If you project "Sorry, but I am only the messenger" or "this speech was not my choice", you will have minimal credibility. If you go on stage and then the first thing you do is to ask for assistance to get the next slide projected, it does not give you any credibility from the start. If you cannot even master a simple technique, how can the rest of your performance have any credibility?

Trustworthiness has to do with your reputation as a medical researcher; however, in my experience, it is amazing the amount of flimsy data and cooked-up stories an audience is willing to forgive. Nevertheless, they have their limits, and your credibility will be lost. Lost credibility in medical science is nearly impossible to restore. So, do not attempt to build a reputation as a speaker on this: One day, the audience will wave the axe.

There is one other aspect of credibility, and that is how to dress. If you are a world-famous doctor, with a long curriculum vitae and prestigious rewards, you can come in jeans and a T-shirt, but for the rest who are still to reach that status, dress appropriately. Find out what the dress code at your specific meeting is. I know that some medical professions have a more artistic dress code but stay in tune. Do not distract the audience with funny or colourful ties, swooping scarves or loud jewellery.

4.1.3
Delivery

Delivery is also important. A great message delivered with a flat voice will not help create the effect you were hoping to create. A good presentation is like a good relationship. A speech is not a performance but rather a relationship you create with an audience. Try to be yourself.

> Speak to one person at a time. Make eye contact with one person at a time for a few seconds instead of scanning the audience.

- Talk as you normally do.
- Speak in short sentences as much as possible; this will help you to be clearer.
- Change the rhythm when you speak.
- I have never heard anybody complain that somebody speaks too slowly; people only complain when someone speaks too fast.
- Emphasise the key points of your lecture by slowing down and focusing on a person in the second row. Tell this person, one to one, what you have to say.

4.2
The Opening Line

Introduce yourself. Even if the chairperson of the session has already introduced you, unless you are sure that everybody in the audience knows who you are, you should always introduce yourself.

Your first slide should be on the screen before you begin

At a scientific session, when presenting your research data, begin as follows:

Good morning [afternoon] ladies and gentlemen, my name is … , I am from … . I am here to present you the results from our trial looking at the relationship between drinking milk and bone fractures in octogenarians.

4.2.1
At an Invited Lecture

Thank the organisers and any key figures for inviting you. But, be aware that it is better to thank no one than to forget the most important one. This can cause major embarrassment, especially in Asia.

4.2.2
How to Get the Attention of the Audience from the Start

For an invited lecture, you can start with a personal anecdote, something about the long-standing relationship between you and the organiser of the meeting or even a pre-prepared anecdote. If you are not creative, you can always look at http://www. anecdote.com.

Know your audience as some anecdotes may hit a wrong note, giving you a bad start, which will completely ruin the rest of your lecture. Anecdotes on any faith or religion, sexuality, age or even hair colour can come back at you like a boomerang.

If you are not the anecdotal type, and many are simply not gifted in this area, there is another simple but effective trick. Just pause for 5 s after your introduction, look around the audience, smile at anybody, take a deep breath and begin. You will see how amazingly easy this is, and it almost always works.

4.3
The Message

The *message* refers to everything a speaker says, both verbally and non-verbally. The message again has different aspects.

Content — Style — Structure

4.3.1
Content

Content is what you present in a lecture. Try to focus on the key elements of what you want to say. A good way to do this is, before you start preparing your lecture, explain to a colleague in only three sentences what you plan to say. If you need more than three sentences to put across the core of your message, you probably will not be able to fit this into a 10-min lecture. Write down what you want the audience to learn or remember from your lecture. This is its core.

- Always decide how much you are going to say. After years of research, you could probably talk for an hour, but you only have 10 min.
- Distinguish the main points from the side issues.
- Do not present conflicting items unless you want to discuss these conflicts.
- Decide the sequence you will use.
- Only use data or arguments that will lead to the conclusion of your lecture.

You will find more on how to structure your content in the chapter on PowerPoint presentations.

There is nothing more embarrassing than being in a lecture session as second or third speaker and hearing one of the speakers before you presenting the main topics of the lecture you have prepared. You are trapped, and there is no way that you can get out of this situation. Of course, it is all your fault; you should have contacted the organisers with a couple of questions:

- Who else is speaking in my session?
- What are their topics?

If you think there might be an overlap, contact your fellow speakers and discuss potential problems. Try to decide who will talk about what.

4.3.2
Style

Style is the manner in which you present the content of your lecture. Styles can vary from informal to very formal. At almost all medical meetings, the formal style is customary. Only invited keynote speakers can have a more informal style, but only to a certain extent. Medicine is a serious business, and doctors take themselves seriously as there is nothing funny about a sick patient or a chronic disease. I address this issue more extensively under the topic of humour elsewhere in this book, but funny YouTube movies, cartoons and jokes will hardly ever improve your invited lecture. Only when you deliver a poor lecture with old and outdated content might your audience be pleased with some light entertainment. If you refuse to be somewhat serious, you might want to put down this book. You are probably very much appreciated as a stand-up comedian but not so much as a serious lecturer.

4.3.3
Structure

Structure is organisation. Every medical lecture should have a structure that is more or less uniform. Especially for those who have less experience, a fixed structure can be helpful in improving presentation. Poorly organised lectures have a reduced impact, and the audience is less likely to accept the data presented.

- *Introduction:* should include an overview of what we already know and the purpose of your lecture in relation to this.
- *Body:* main points and data that support your message and conclusion.
- *Conclusion:* follows from the points you have presented in the body. Never present a conclusion that is not supported by the data.

Another important point to consider is your allowed speaking time. Going overtime is always perceived by the audience, as well as your fellow speakers, as impolite and annoying. This behaviour can completely ruin a session. Other speakers will have less time for their lecture because of you, and there will not be any time left for questions and answers. A good chairperson will make sure the speakers keep to their time, but unfortunately there are only a few chairpersons with enough authority to stop a speaker mid-presentation.

How to be a good chairperson is discussed elsewhere in this book.

4.4
Audience

At a medical meeting, the audience is almost always made up of physicians, which makes it both easy and difficult. It is easy because one can assume that they all have a medical background, which helps with communication. Many items are known and need no further explanation; therefore, one can concentrate on the key points of the lecture that add to this mutual knowledge. It is difficult because the level of knowledge of a medical audience can vary greatly. Some are juniors who need more explanation, while others will find your presentation too basic. Always do a proper audience analysis if you are an invited speaker. Ask the organisers about this before you start preparing to be sure that you will give the right lecture to the right audience. Make a list of specific questions and send them to the organisers. If you are asked to talk about the same topic at a number of medical meetings in the same year, be aware that you will not be addressing the same audience you met just 6 months ago.

4.5
Communication Channels

There are a lot of channels you can use to communicate with an audience. Your lecture as you have prepared it is only one aspect, but without proper use of the other communication channels, it will not work. The more channels you use, the better.

4.5.1
Non-Verbal Communication

Non-verbal communication is all those things that add to the (often subconscious) impression the audience has of you – how they feel about you, not necessarily related your lecture. Some people are natural masters in non-verbal communication; they have what we call *charisma*. Even if most of what they say is a slight variation from the truth, they are almost always saved by their charisma. I would not advise you to do the same for your scientific presentations; the chances of your colleagues forgiving you based on your charisma alone are slim.

Non-verbal communications are things like gestures, facial expressions, body movements and postures:

- *Gestures* can help, but too many of them can also be annoying and distracting. Highlighting what you want to say by using your hands can work. Lecturers who stand like a wooden statue, without any movement of the arms, do not demonstrate any passion or feeling for the message they want to get across. However, waving your arms all the time, like you are dancing, does not do you any favours at all. Raising your arms every now and then can have its psychological benefits. Using appropriate gestures can make your presence appear larger and can help to assert authority over others.
- *Facial expressions* were less important in the past, but currently at larger medical meetings a speaker is often projected in the background on a large screen. Look relaxed, smile and do not look angry. Show that you are happy to be where you are, even if you really want to be somewhere else.
- *Body movements* are the same as gestures. Do not stand like a wooden statue, but again, too much movement can be distracting. If you are invited for a more personal lecture, like a keynote lecture or an honorary lecture, it could work in your favour to step to the side of the lectern to deliver your talk. This is a trick you often see with politicians. If you want to do this, you will have to plan in advance (see Sect. 5.2 of Chap. 5). Be sure to have enough space to move around on the

stage, and that you are not lost in the wilderness of stage flowers. Of course, you need a wireless microphone and a remote slide control. You will also need to make sure that you can see a monitor to avoid having to look back all the time to check that the right slide is projected. This direct contact with the audience, while still being in full control, can in my experience have a major impact on your presentation. However, pick your moments carefully, it should not be your signature style; it depends on the element of surprise.

- *Posture* is important; try to create the impression that you are tall. Stand straight, with your chest out and shoulders down. If you are not so tall, wear some special shoes. Ask the room technician, before the session starts, for a platform to stand on behind the lectern. Most lecture halls have such an aid available if you ask for this in time. Do ask for a platform when you step behind the lectern to start your presentation; this will make you look even smaller.

Some years ago, I was invited to a pleasant medical meeting; the hotel that housed the lecture hall was right next to a beautiful sunny beach. I was sitting in the audience when the following scene unfolded:

The invited speaker had cancelled his participation at the last minute, and he had sent his research fellow to give his presentation. As she had done all the scientific research and was a native English speaker, this would not be a big problem. The chairperson explained the situation and asked the replacement, Dr. Green, to come to the stage. As the chairperson spoke about "he" and "him" and not "her" and "she", it was obvious that he was not aware of the gender of the replacement. Dr. Green took the stage: high heels, short dress and large sunglasses on top of her head. Dr. Green was also of small stature, despite her high shoes. As she disappeared behind the lectern, the chairperson again asked if Dr. Green was in the room. Two hands moved up to pull the microphone all the way down behind the lectern. "Yes, I am here", the sunglasses answered. All the way through her lecture, the only thing you could see was some wild curly hair, with those huge sunglasses on top, moving while she spoke. This lecture is now known as the famous "sunglass lecture". The audience was dumbfounded, but this had little to do with her lecture content.

4.5.2
Verbal Communication

Verbal communication is again an important aspect of how your lecture is perceived. There are two things to consider here: tone of your voice and variations in pitch and volume.

- *Tone of your voice* is more or less a fixed element. Trying to change it is difficult. You are a soprano, a bass, or some level in between: That is what you are. There are things that you can improve. If you have a nasal voice, try to talk more with your lips and in the proximal part of your oral cavity. Articulate, do not swallow the words; it is better to exaggerate your speech than to try to be overly natural.

- *Variations in pitch and volume* will make listening to your lecture much more pleasant. Most speakers, especially those who are nervous or less experienced, speak too fast and monotonously. **It is almost impossible to speak too slowly.** Try to take a break between items; often, 2 s is enough to keep the attention of the audience. Try to accentuate with the volume of your voice. They work best after a short 2 s break. Do not let your voice tail, which is to start each sentence in a strong manner but then allowing your voice to sag or tail off.

Practise finishing your sentences in a strong manner.

4.6
How to Keep Your Audience Focussed

Cross-references. Make cross-references to things you have said or discussed earlier in your talk.

Transitions. Do not jump from one item to another without connecting them. Make logical transitions during your lecture.

Repetition. Repeat themes or items, which you have discussed earlier in your talk, but in a slightly different way. Remember that you have to repeat a message at least three times during your talk before people will remember it: Tell them what you will tell them, tell them and tell them what you told them.

Rhetorical questions. You can incorporate one or more rhetorical questions in your talk and let the answer be the start of the next paragraph in your lecture.

Internal summary. Pause at major transitions and recapitulate what has been said before you move on to the next item of your lecture.

4.7
Noise

Noise can be distracting, especially when you are inexperienced. You must get used to two types of noises: external and internal.

- *External noise* includes sounds from the audience, people talking, people walking in and out, mobile phones, poor acoustics, air conditioning and many other things. You should try to ignore them completely. A room can be too hot or too cold, or your slides may not be clearly visible. Ignore it or try to make it work for you: "On the next, just as a blurred slide, you will see … ," or in a cold room. "I have never been in a room as cold as this; there are penguins sitting here in the first row."
- *Internal noise* – If a speaker is unclear or confused about how to express his or her message, this can be avoided by good preparation.

If you are known to have trouble with internal noise despite good preparation and using all the channels of communication, verbal and non-verbal, you can use the ultimate solution.

As an experienced speaker, I find it difficult to advise this, but you can also read your lecture from a piece of paper. Is this as bad as public-speaking gurus make out? I think a well-prepared lecture with good content read from a manuscript is always better than a confused and unclear lecture learned by heart. This is especially true of scientific presentations for which time, content and precise data are important; having a piece of paper with what you want to say can be helpful. Never condemn anybody who presents from paper: A lecture is not a play; it is all about transmitting information and knowledge.

4.8
How to Finish

You can give a fine lecture with nice content and finish within the time limit and still ruin it in the last moment.

Do not just stop and leave them confused.

This is similar to a classical concert when the audience is in doubt if silence means that it is finished and their applause can start. You do not want to be that cultural barbarian who alone starts to applaud when there is still more to come. I hate these moments.

Do not say "*That's it,*" "*That's the end,*" or "*I'm finished*".

Never offer to answer questions if there is a chairperson; it is the role of the chairperson, not you, to ask for questions.

Inviting questions by the lecturer is rude; you should never do this.

Never walk off the stage before the chairperson has finished the discussion and gives you the sign that you may step down.

Do not show that applause slide at the end; it is embarrassing to beg for applause.

Just keep it simple and finish by saying; "Thank you very much for your attention."

4.9
General Rules for Every Presenter

- Always make yourself known to the chairperson before the session starts.
- Ask if there are any changes in the programme.
- If you are replacing a presenter who could not make it, bring this to the chairperson's attention before the session starts.
- Make yourself familiar with the audiovisual system in the room. Ask the room assistant to briefly explain the function of the buttons on the lectern to you.

The best way to handle your (time) planning is to talk with the persons chairing the session beforehand and to ask them how they are planning to organise the session.

Is there going to be time for questions after each lecture or questions at the end of the session? The latter is often the case when all presentations are on one specific topic. If you have been allocated 10 min including questions from the audience, ask if you can have the 10 min without questions if you need more time. However, this is almost never possible. The chairperson is in charge of the session and will decide how the session is run, so always find this out before you start. In case of a late cancellation, the chairperson can give each speaker more time, and it is good to know this ahead of time. Usually, a good chairperson will make a speaker aware if the time limit has been exceeded. There are speakers who simply choose to ignore this, but this is not well received, to say the least. Some meetings have a more depersonalised approach to ensuring that speakers obey their time slots. There are systems with warning lights; green is "speak", orange is "wrap it up" (normally meaning 2 min to go) and red is "stop". Some sessions also project a timer at the bottom of the presentation screen showing the remaining speaking time. Both systems are sometimes combined with an arrangement in which the microphone is automatically turned off at the end of the individual time slot. The first time I saw this system not all of the presenters actually noticed that their sound was turned off and carried on as if nothing had happened – in a loud voice. There is nothing more frustrating and embarrassing than having your presentation stopped before you come to your conclusions. The years of work and the expectations of how your colleagues will react to your scientific findings are lost, not to mention the financial investment you and your department have made for you to be on that stage.

Not keeping to your time slot is therefore highly unadvisable; it can and should be avoided at all times.

Key Points

- Talk to the chairperson about your time slot.
- Find out how the session is organised.
- Ten minutes gross speaking time is 7–8 min net.
- Exceeding the time limit is a major flaw.

4.10
Summary

- So far, we have discussed the ways to communicate with an audience. For your lecture, you should use them all.
- Go over all the discussed items one by one and try to think about which areas you can improve. Only by bearing all these elements in mind will you be in a position to create the perfect speech.
- Prepare your talk, rehearse and time yourself as many times as possible until you feel comfortable and it becomes part of you.

- Some tape their talk or video it. Listening or looking back, you will recognise your weaker points of communication. Personally, I have never tried this, but I know that some swear by it.
- Ask your colleagues to listen to your presentation and discuss your lecture with them before going to the meeting.

What I do when I have an important lecture is try to work on the rhythm and flow of its delivery. I go through my lecture in my head while I walk outdoors through a field or on the beach, increasing and decreasing my walking speed and at the same time increasing and decreasing the virtual presentation in my head. I just hammer it in and make it part of me. Lecture and self are now unified. It really works for me, and maybe it can also work for you.

4.11
How to Overcome Stage Fright

Butterflies, trembling, voice quivers, shortness of breath, sweaty palms, pacing and so forth.
Everybody has experienced at least one of these when on stage. I certainly have not met anybody who has not. Some still experience stage fright even after hundreds of lectures, while others seem to overcome it. Having some tension (adrenalin) before you start is good; it helps you think and concentrate. However, it should not take over your performance.
The best way to deal with the fear of public speaking is to control the situation and make stress your friend.

4.11.1
Failure

Failure is what everybody fears: embarrassment, making a fool out of yourself. The better prepared your lecture is, the less chance there is that you will fail. Prepare and discuss your doubts and uncertainties before you go to the meeting so that they become the strong points of your lecture. It is no problem if you skip a key point; nobody will realise it. You are just creating an opportunity for somebody to ask a question that is easy for you to answer.

4.11.2
Environment

Environment is the lecture hall. Arrive early and walk around; sit and observe the audience's perspective. Go and stand behind the lectern and get used to the set-up.

4.11.3
Audience

The audience is for many the greatest fear. Remember that the audience is your friend; they are on your side. Have you ever gone to a lecture hoping the lecturer would fail? Of course not. As long as you bring something of value, you will be fine. Be in the lecture hall when the audience comes in; welcome friends if you see them and engage in some small talk. Ask your friends to sit somewhere in front; you can pretend that you are having your own mini-meeting. Or, imagine that you are having a conversation with people in the audience. Do not speak *to* an audience but *with* an audience. If you can make that personal connection, it will help to overcome your fear, and your lecture will be much more appreciated.

4.11.4
Rehearsal

Rehearsal is to make your lecture part of you. Know your material and prepare, prepare, prepare. If you are confident about what you are going to do, if you know the details of the material that you are going to present, that will take away a lot of your stage fright. You can practise your lecture in front of a mirror or a friend, but this will not be nearly as effective as being well prepared.

Although all doctors are strong believers that medication can cure all problems, I do not know of any medication (e.g. beta-blockers) that will help you get over your fear of public speaking. The most it will do is make you dizzy, sleepy, numb and a poor lecturer. Things that might help are breathing exercises like yoga, simple stretching exercises or a quick walk in the fresh air 30 min before the session starts. A light breakfast or lunch, no carbonated drinks and no alcohol should help.

A highly renowned speaker gave me two tips, which I have never tried, but they might work for you:

- Eating bananas before your lecture might help you to relax.
- Imagine the audience naked.

My personal tip is

Use positive thinking: "Yes, I can", "Is there any reason I can't? No!"

But, take care not to become arrogant as this will irritate any audience.

4.11.5
Classic Fears

We finally have to discuss the following:
Fear of fainting. This is unlikely to happen unless you have a real medical problem.

Fear of boring the audience. This will not happen if you present interesting material, especially if you use an enthusiastic voice. Audiences like passionate speakers who show that they believe in their message.

Fear of your mind going blank. I have seen it happen. Do not panic; just take a short pause and a sip of water (which is never used by any speaker). Pick up where you left off or skip this item and move on to the next.

Fear of being judged. Any presenter who shows passion and who believes in his or her presentation will never be judged negatively.

> Three basic tips to help in your struggle with stage fright.

- *Arrive early.* Arriving at the last minute is stressful even for experienced speakers. Survey the surroundings, make a trip to the restroom, organise your thoughts and check the facilities.
- *Eat lightly.* Do not intake alcohol and eat nothing that can give you an upset stomach.
- *Look for friends.* Their presence will often help you relax.

However, the best way to kill stage fright is to speak frequently, so small local meetings are an excellent way to work on your performance and deal with stage fright.

4.12
Handling Questions and Answers

Answering questions is something many speakers fear; nevertheless, it is a great opportunity to impress your audience with your (prepared) knowledge and to repeat the important points of your lecture.

How to be in charge of what is happening during questions and answers

- If you are asked a question from the audience, always ask the speaker to use the microphone if he or she is not already doing so (you are in charge).
- If the questioner speaks unclearly, bend forward a little, put your right hand behind your ear and ask the questioner to repeat the question (you are in charge).
- Paraphrase the question before answering it; this helps you understand the question and gives you extra time to think about the answer.
- If you do not know the answer, say so. Do not try to make one up. You can say that you will find out and let the questioner know later. Or say, "That's an interesting point. I'll have to think about it. Maybe we should discuss this off-line".
- Never get into a discussion with the audience.
- Never put a question down as stupid; no audience will like that. (Do not say: "Did you sleep during my lecture?" or "Are you a doctor?")

- If a question is perfect for you to reemphasize one of the key points of your lecture, compliment the person who has posed the question ("Thank you for this question"). You will have a friend for life.

4.13
Being a Chairperson

Being a chairperson is not merely an honourable position, as some believe. As a meeting organiser, I was often asked by colleagues if I had a chairmanship for them in one of the sessions as they fancied holding an important position. Being chairperson really is an important role and requires good preparation. You do not just sit there and announce the next speaker. You and, if applicable, your co-chairperson are in charge of the session. You see to it that every speaker has his or her allocated time, that nobody goes over time, and that there is ample space in the session for questions and answers. You will decide when and how many questions should be asked. You would have prepared some questions (if there are none from the audience) to start and to stimulate a discussion. You are the one who can take a session to a higher level.

Obligations of a Chairperson

- To be prepared. For this, he or she has to read all abstracts in advance.
- To be in the room to welcome the speakers before the session starts.
- To put the speakers at ease.
- To act as time keeper.
- To announce the speakers. For an invited lecture, this should be done with a personal note about the speaker.
- To lead or start the period for questions and answers.
- To end the session.

Time management is important. As a chairperson, you should clearly tell each speaker the amount of time he or she has before the session starts. In addition, tell them that after X minutes you will give a sign to let them know that they should wrap up the presentation. At the beginning, after opening the session, the chairperson should again say how much time each speaker has. Announce that the speaker will be asked to stop when his or her time is up, so the audience will not be surprised. Be strict with all or with nobody, but treat every lecturer the same way.

And finally …

It is all about the lecturers, not about the chairperson, although I have at times seen otherwise, with the chairperson the most prominent speaker in the room. This is like a football referee who also takes the penalty shot.

Special Medical Presentations

5

Contents

5.1
Presenting a Workshop

In addition to holding a lecture, you may be asked to give a workshop. This raises a crucial point that many have a tendency to forget:

> A workshop is not a lecture for a small group.

A workshop is an interactive exchange of knowledge. The duration of a workshop is always longer than that of a lecture, most are 30–60 min, and the structure is different. The most important role of the workshop presenter is to create an ambiance in which questions and answers flow naturally. It is a combination of education and determining the audience's gaps in knowledge. The best workshops are those that offer lively interaction and an open forum without a prefixed rigid structure, which is in stark contrast to a lecture, for which organisation is the most important element. To be able to hold such a workshop, the presenter should, first and foremost, be an authority in the

J.A. Reekers, *Presenting at Medical Meetings*,
DOI: 10.1007/978-3-642-12408-2_5, © Springer-Verlag Berlin Heidelberg 2010

field. However, that is not to say that the presenters come away from the workshop without having learned something themselves. On the contrary, over the years, I have experienced that, in a good workshop, new learning is the case.

In a lecture, you can hide behind your performance and presentation; this is not true of a workshop. You should be in the vulnerable position of authority, open to questions from participants and safe in the knowledge of being on top of your chosen subject. A workshop should be a mixture of educational interaction, group feeling and individual endeavour.

The following items should be considered when planning a workshop:

- Format
- Materials and content
- Technical support
- Presentation
- Workload
- Educational tools
- Feedback

5.1.1
Format

The format of a workshop should be informal and personal. You therefore need a room that accommodates this. It is virtually impossible to give a workshop in a main auditorium. If this is suggested by the meeting organisers, protest firmly or simply decline. It is a waste of time and effort, and you will only be frustrated in the end. Thirty people in a 1,200-seat auditorium do not create the right ambiance for a fruitful workshop. Asking people to come and sit in the first few rows is, at least in my experience, never successful. Should this lead to a refusal, this then creates a considerable physiological gap, and your authority is jeopardised from the beginning. Workshops with a maximum of around 50 people are often the most successful. For small workgroups of up to 20 people, a U-shaped table can be put in place. For larger audiences, theatre style is recommended. Make sure that everybody is able to see and hear you, and that there is enough space for you to walk around should you intend to do so. Never give a workshop from behind a lectern as this will create distance between you and the participants. To reiterate, a workshop is not a lecture for a small group. There are many ways to create an open and informal atmosphere; just select what best fits your personality. Remember, the workshop should have a natural feel to it. Some dress informally to achieve this, but you can also stroll around or casually perch on a table.

One way I sometimes try to create a good atmosphere for a workshop is to make sure I am in the room as the participants are entering. I make light conversation with some of them when they are seated, asking how their meeting is progressing and what they think of the meeting so far. When it is time to start, I introduce myself and begin by saying, "This is a workshop, which means that you have to work before you can shop" or "It is our workshop, not my workshop". I then encourage them to interact by interrupting me any time they have a question or when they think I am talking nonsense. Then, I take of my jacket, and if I am wearing a tie, I also take that off. That is probably as far as the disrobing should go. Such an introduction, which differentiates this format from that of a standard lecture, is the best way to capture their undivided attention. You are now the focus. I then ask standard questions like, "Is anyone here already experienced in the topic at hand?" This way I can identify those who can be involved in a discussion later.

For a small group, using a microphone is not ideal; it creates a barrier and blocks discussions as the audience will also need microphones. For larger groups, audio support is fine, but this should not be too loud.

If there are questions, always repeat the question back to the audience or rephrase it to better fit with your educational goals. Answer directly to the person, and do not give a general answer. If possible, try to interact with some of the more experienced attendees you have by now identified in the audience.

A workshop must have a flexible structure and address the needs and questions of the audience.

5.1.2
Materials and Content

Regarding materials and content, a golden rule for any workshop is to remain focussed; do not attempt to tackle the whole subject. Keep it simple and do not stray from the point. Showing off about how great and academic you are is not the right approach to an interactive workshop.

Start with some simple examples to get everybody on board and then proceed to a higher level. For instance, if a particular technique is being taught at a workshop, do not begin with a showcase of your most fantastic results. The materials to bring to a workshop depend on the chosen topic. A workshop on cases or techniques requires different materials compared to one on pharmaceuticals. The easiest way to present your supporting materials is using a PowerPoint presentation. But, be aware that you run the risk of heavily depending on your materials and that your workshop will turn into a formal lecture. Any materials, from medical demo devices to handouts, PowerPoints and videos can be used as long as they stimulate interactive discussions and carry a message.

5.1.3
Technical Support

Technical support very much depends on what you are planning to do. We have been overwhelmed with all kinds of technology – PowerPoint, interactive blackboards and online interactive Internet programmes – which can all be used during a workshop. Sometimes, however, a simple flip chart is more than enough to produce an effective workshop. Remember that, just as with formal presentations, "less is more". Whatever technology you are planning to use, always check and re-check it ahead of time, make sure you rehearse and that somebody is available to help in case of any technical problems. Failing techniques will be detrimental to your workshop, and you will have a difficult time regaining your audience's attention.

5.1.4
Presentation

To initiate your presentation, briefly introduce yourself and provide your credentials. You want to establish yourself as a professional and an authority but do not brag about or linger on this point. Better yet, weave this information into your presentation. People are here to learn, not to massage your ego. Most important, thank the attendees for coming. Make this sincere rather than routine. Single out a few individuals who you recognise and let them know you appreciate their attendance.

There are a couple of standard points not to forget, although they are not applicable to every situation.

- A good ice-breaker will relax everyone in the room, including you.
- Involve the audience. Ask them why they came and what they are hoping to achieve.
- Tell a story, make a point – tell a story, make a point.
- Observe the behaviour in the room; try to identify the "quick" learners, the "stragglers", the "quiet ones" or the "troublemakers", who always have something to say.
- Keep the presentation focussed. If one particularly animated soul likes the sound of his or her own voice or brings up a side issue, be sure to address that individual or issue and let the individual know that it is outside the scope of the workshop, but that you would be glad to talk to them about it later.
- Make eye contact with individuals.
- Engage the audience. The best way to do this is to ask questions and ask for a show of hands; such "have you ever … " questions help the audience relate to you and your topic. Initiate a conversation.
- Another way to engage your audience is through the idea of exclusivity. Humans do not want to be left out of a good thing. Tell them that you are about to unveil a new fact or inside tip that you have never before shared with anybody.
- Create infotainment, which is combining information with light entertainment.
- Keep the enthusiasm and trim the detail.
- By adding context, you can bring an emotional quality to the statistics that you are presenting and frame the numbers in a way that gives them added meaning.

For example, if you have a workshop on amputations due to diabetic foot problems, you can present the figures in a scientific way. However, you can also recalculate that worldwide a limb is going to be amputated due to diabetic foot problems every minute. "Ladies and gentlemen", you then say, "This means that during this 1-h workshop, 60 limbs will have been amputated worldwide". This is just the kind of context that grabs the audience's attention and will make your workshop something that they will remember long after it is over.

5.1.5
Workload

A good workshop should not contain too much information. If you are able to communicate a few key points, the workshop can already be deemed a success. Your workload depends on you. You can base a presentation on one or many main themes. The latter will largely be steered by the audience by means of questions and discussion points, thus requiring their enthusiasm and active involvement. However, this can be a tricky format that is best suited to presentations to students; their thirst for knowledge drives their interest and curiosity. Experienced professionals do not always respond well to such prompts or scenarios. Although I would advise you to incorporate one leading theme only in a standard workshop, you need to be prepared for different situations due to the unpredictable nature of the sessions. So, as is the case with formal presentations, you should rehearse in front of a small audience at home. Always bring more material than is needed and organise your presentation tool (i.e. PowerPoint) in such a way that allows it to be scrolled forward or backward according to audience feedback. This further supports the need for a flexibly structured workshop directed by the needs and questions of the audience.

5.1.6
Presentation Tools

For a workshop, you can choose many different presentation tools. I have even seen a workshop at which the presenter brought nothing but himself. He started a conversation with a member of the audience and extended it to the whole group, ending with a lively, interactive group of participants. This is the most difficult format, and I would not promote it here, although it is the highest form of communication. The easiest and most reliable tool is PowerPoint (please see Chap. 3). It is important to remember that PowerPoint should not be used as an autocue tool as this will block interaction with the workshop participants. However, if you talk about medical devices or specific techniques, you can bring demo devices for people to familiarise them and for them to handle. You could also bring models so the participants can work on them; this is usually referred to as a *hands-on workshop*, which also follows the rules outlined in the previous discussion.

Simple tools like a flip chart can also be helpful, especially to note the thoughts and ideas of the group as a starting point for discussion. Employ the most appropriate methods, which may not necessarily be the most sophisticated. Participants have come to see and hear you, not the latest presentation techniques. Always remember, a good workshop is informal, and the flow of information should be two way.

5.1.7
Feedback

To continuously improve your workshop performance, audience input is essential. Try to evaluate your workshop immediately after you have finished, making notes on what went well and what went wrong, which topics initiated good interaction and discussion and which did not. Ask the participants to fill out evaluation forms and, if the opportunity arises, speak to one of the active participants directly after the workshop and note his or her remarks. Immediate feedback, when the iron is still hot, is the best way to improve your next workshop.

Summary

- A workshop is not a lecture.
- Try to create an informal atmosphere that encourages two-way flow of information.
- Let the audience determine the direction of the workshop.
- Do not attempt to impress anybody with your authority.
- Less is more.

5.2
The Al Gore Presentation

Those of you who have seen the 2006 Al Gore movie *An Inconvenient Truth* must have been impressed by his presentation style and the blending of speech and visual content. As a medical doctor, you can only do this kind of presentation if you are an invited keynote speaker and a recognised personality in your medical specialty. A presentation like this is a highlight in your career and should not be repeated every year. I have done it once when I was invited to give the 2008 Dotter lecture at the Society of Interventional Radiology in Washington, D.C. It needs a lot of preparation and experience, and I would not advise it to anybody who feels insecure on stage. For those who think it is their time, I reveal some basic tricks.

5.2.1
Full Body Exposure

Full-body exposure is when you stand in front of an audience and not behind a lectern to give your lecture. Just stepping to the side of the lectern is not full-body exposure. When your position is higher than the audience and they can see you from head to toe, that is the real thing. You need a stage floor where you can walk around and focus on different sections of the audience. However, the audience must be able to see you at all times. If they do not see you but only hear you, they will lose interest. Make sure that your walking path is free of obstacles so you do not stumble over anything. If so, you will certainly be remembered for that but not for your lecture. Clothing is important; wear something neutral that does not distract. Whether you should wear your jacket open or closed, with one or more buttons unbuttoned, or with only the top button unbuttoned, I have no idea. Al Gore in *An Inconvenient Truth* did not wear a tie and had one button closed, but he is the former vice-president of the United States. This way of presenting can be powerful if you do it right, but if you do it wrong it is really wrong.

5.2.2
Blending Speech and Visual Content

Blending speech and visual content is something that adds to the magic of this kind of presentation. First, you need a good small wireless microphone (test whether it works). Then, you need one or two small monitors that will show you the actual slide presented behind you. These monitors should be positioned in front of the stage or at the front edge. You can camouflage them with some flowers. They should be large enough that you can see and read them from your position on the stage so that you do not have to turn around to look at your slides all the time. Now, here is the second part of the magic: a small wireless remote to bring your slides forward or, when needed, backward. It should be small enough to fit into your hand so it is not obvious. So, you walk around with your wireless microphone, look to the audience, peek at one of the monitors in front of you, and move your slides forward with your wireless remote. The audience will be flabbergasted, and your lecture will be remembered forever.

5.3
Medical Presentation for Non-Medical Audience

The medical presentation for a non-medical audience is one of the most difficult things to do. You really have to prepare carefully, and you should be absolutely clear about the message you want to get across. Do not send a message that can be understood in different ways or, worse, a message with an open end. When presenting for an medical audience, you can presume a certain basic knowledge that gives you the opportunity to take bigger steps, to talk about more detailed information and to leave question marks in your talk. This is not true for a non-medical audience. You have to take small steps and be specific but not detailed. Anything you say will be acknowledged as coming from the authority. You lose that authority by being vague or by patronising the audience. A non-medical audience does not have the reference to judge and balance the importance of every part of your lecture. You have to take this in consideration when you start preparing your talk.

Some Basic Rules

- Give no more than one to two messages.
- Give no detailed information.
- Do not presume any medical reference.
- Do not use medical slang.
- Repeat the main messages four to six times in a different form to drive them home.
- Keep distance; you are the authority.
- Do not patronise.
- Use simple slides and illustrations; they may not be used to this kind of visual information.
- Only use a few slides that support your main message.

— Always start your talk by explaining why it is specifically you who are standing before them. Do not say: "I was asked to give this speech". Say: "As a specialist in the field of … , it is for me a great pleasure … ."
— If you talk to a group representing a certain patient interest or disease, be clear to tell them that you know who they are and why they are there.
— Make contact and determine your position and theirs regarding the knowledge about the topic.

5.3.1
Lighting

Normally during a medical lecture, the lights in the lecture hall are dimmed during the lecture, with a spot on the lecturer, so it is easier to see the PowerPoint illustrations. For a non-medical audience, I would advise you to have the lecture hall more illuminated so that participants will still experience themselves as part of a group and not isolated in the dark. You will see that a non-medical audience almost always has a few leaders, those who will ask the questions, and these individuals need to be recognised by the others. You should not create a non-natural atmosphere by putting them in the dark.

Secondly, you need to see the reactions of your audience to be able to modify the pace of your lecture. If some start to disconnect during your lecture, you will see that and can target them by focussing on them.

5.3.2
Timing

Time is usually not too strict as you are often the only speaker. They all came to see YOU. A lecture of no more than 30 min to a non-medical audience is probably optimal. After 30 min, their attention will decrease.

Ten minutes is too short; remember that you are the lecturer they came to see.

A good way to keep the full attention of the audience is to divide your talk into 10-min segments, with a crescendo at the end of each part. You then pause for a few seconds; you can than take a drink of water, look around and continue, for example, with "Okay, let's go on". Three 10-min talks are easier to digest than one 30-min talk.

Always give a clear summary of what you have covered.

Thank the audience for their attention or for the opportunity to be able to give the lecture.

Leave ample time for questions. This is to check if your messages have arrived and to be able to correct misunderstandings.

Do not say: "You got it completely wrong"; say "This is not exactly what I wanted to tell".

When you are done with your lecture and the questions, do not just leave the room, but be around so that those who were not stepping to the microphone are also able to ask you their questions.

The Social Environment of a Medical Meeting

6

Contents

When attending a larger medical meeting, especially for the first time, it is difficult not to be overwhelmed by your impressions and the sheer amount of information offered. You are entering a new and glamorous world where you first have to find your own bearing. Are you coming to learn new things, to get an educational update, to hear about the latest science, to meet friends or to become part of the old boys' speakers' network? There are some basic rules and principles for everybody to understand and to maintain. It starts as early as registration with your badge and congress bag.

6.1
Registration

Registering for a meeting is not a simple formality; there are serious financial implications attached to how and when you register. In general, one can say that the earlier you register, the cheaper it is. These reductions can amount to up to 50% for the "early birds". So, always register early, at least when a sponsoring company is not paying for you. Being invited by industry was rather normal for many years; however, recent changes in legislation, both in Europe and the United States, now forbid this practice. Sometimes, it can be cheaper to first become a member of the organising society to be eligible for the reduced

J.A. Reekers, *Presenting at Medical Meetings*,
DOI: 10.1007/978-3-642-12408-2_6, © Springer-Verlag Berlin Heidelberg 2010

member-only fees. This is especially true if you are planning on regularly visiting this specific meeting in the future. Other benefits of being a society member, like the journal and e-mail alerts, are then free as well. There are often special rates for nurses, juniors or trainees, which can also bring considerable discounts, if applicable.

There are ways to avoid proper registration, but I had always believed these to be mere rumours, thinking that no self-respecting doctor would want to be exposed as a fraud. As badge control is now standard at most larger meetings, attending without a proper badge, which gives you access to the lecture halls and technical exhibition, requires a preconceived plan. I now know, after being around for all these years at medical meetings, that people do under-register.

Under-registration is, for example, to register as a participating nurse at a much lower fee when you are actually a full physician. Of course, to register as a trainee is self-limiting unless you spend a fortune on cosmetic surgery, which does not sound cost-effective to me in the long run. A real underhanded plan is to claim that you have lost your badge when in reality you gave it to a colleague with whom you share the registration fee 50/50. With both under-registration and all other tricks, you will not receive your continuous medical education (CME) points (see the next section), which are vital for your professional education status at board re-certification. Finally, this is not as clever as it looks at first glance.

At larger meetings, there are often separate registration desks for invited speakers and guests. This will save you from queueing.

6.1.1
The Badge

The badge is your stamp, your identity for the outside world; it tells who you are and your association or affiliation. By wearing the badge, you show why you are there. But, it can also reveal your position on the medical ladder. It can show if you are a member or even one step higher, a fellow of the organising society. And, you will see that there are badges with tags for donators (to the research foundation), faculty, president and meeting chair and badges for past presidents, honorary members, gold medallists and many more. These are all ranks that might be waiting for you if your ego and ambition are big enough. In this way, the badge can be more than an ID; it can be a means of differentiating you from the other "ordinary" participants, or it can be a stigma for those who never moved up the ladder. It also distinguishes doctors from industry representatives, often called *industry partners*. By the way, without these partners there would be no badge at all as it would not be possible to organise any medical meeting of any size. But, I will talk about the industry partners and how to deal with them in the section on faculty. Wear your badge, often with an advertisement cord, in a casual way around your neck when you are at the meeting.

A major mistake, as a novice participant, is to keep wearing the badge when you are on public transport on your way back to your hotel. You even can see participants wearing their badges in the bar when they are having a beer at night. You might want to avoid doing that so you do not look like a lonely loser looking for company.

Some badges contain more than your name; they can have special bar codes that are scanned on entering or leaving a lecture hall. This is to provide you with your CME credits after the meeting is over. This is only seen at bigger and more serious meetings for which

CME accreditation is not already provided in the congress bag when you arrive. For some, the last is a good incentive to adjust their educational programme plans to include the local pleasures. But, there is more about these pleasures in the next chapter.

6.1.2
The Congress Bag

The congress bag is an important sign of how important or prestigious the meeting is. A small plastic bag should raise alarm bells, while a bag that can also be used after the meeting is a positive sign. Colour matters; for instance, a yellow bag is easy to recognise but not something a respectable doctor wants to carry around. On the other hand, a nice and recognisable congress bag can be used to build a corporate identity or to create a "family" feeling. Most bags, however, are "one-day stands" to be left at the meeting or dumped in the hotel when the meeting is over. It is rare that one takes a bag home to re-use or to show that you have been to that particular meeting. Novices usually take the first three bags home.

Some years ago, shortly after 9/11, I was at a small meeting in Hamburg with a group of Dutch colleagues. We all had the same travel plans. At this industry-sponsored meeting, we received a rather huge rucksack as a congress bag. Because we travelled home as a group, together with the local industry partners from the organising company, nobody dumped this rucksack as there was no opportunity to do so. We all faithfully carried our congress bags with us as hand luggage onto the plane except for one who managed to get rid of it behind a large planter at the airport just before boarding the plane. It was a few weeks later that I was visited by one of the company representatives, who told me the rest of the story. Just after we had taken off, a worried passenger noticed the huge suspicious rucksack behind the planter and alarmed airport security. The whole airport was evacuated, and all incoming flights were directed to another airport while all outgoing flights were cancelled. The rucksack was removed by a special bomb squad and detonated outside the airport. The company, whose name prominently appeared on the rucksack, was visited by police and received an official warning. This is probably the biggest impact a congress bag has ever had.

In every bag, there are the usual items, which can be divided into three categories:

- A congress book and a programme overview with programme outline and floor plan. Both are practical and should be kept.
- An evaluation form, which should be returned at the end of the meeting. Always tell the organisers your anonymous, unpolished opinion. Although no congress organiser will take this seriously, this form is obligatory for a meeting to receive CME points. It is also a good way to get rid of all your frustrations about the meeting, like not being invited to a company dinner.
- The majority of the content is advertisements, invitations to visit a booth and to receive a nice gift, announcements for upcoming meetings, a pen that might not work and some writing paper for your notes.

As an old congress veteran, I have to give you one important warning. *Never put any personal items* like your wallet, mobile phone or computer *in the congress bag*. If you lose your bag, it will be virtually impossible to find it again amongst the thousands of other identical bags.

Now that you have a badge, a congress bag, a congress book and a programme outline with floor plan, your meeting can start.

However, there is still one important thing I would advise you to do: Make a **meeting agenda** or timetable. Make a day-by-day plan of which lectures you want to hear, which workshops you want to attend, which lectures you yourself have to hold and which social and private appointments you have. This diary is probably the easiest way to get the most out of your medical meeting.

Now, choose your first lecture and let it all happen.

6.2
Attending a Lecture

Again, how to attend a lecture is something that has to be learned. You do not walk into a lecture room and just sit anywhere but have to strategically plan your approach. The chairs at the back do nicely for some much needed shuteye; proceed to the front if you either want to learn something or be seen attending this particular lecture, and position yourself close to a microphone if you plan to ask any questions. For the novice, a place right in the middle is best as it allows you to observe how other, more experienced congress tigers behave.

6.2.1
Mobile Phones

Mobile phones should of course always be turned off or at least be placed on silent mode. This basic rule of respect vis-à-vis the presenters, however, has been much devalued of late. In more southern European countries, it seems normal not only to leave your mobile phone on during a presentation but also to answer all calls while sitting in the lecture room. The excuse some use is that they are head of a department and that they should always be available to make important medical decisions. I do not know if this counts as "telemedicine", but I think it is just impolite. By the way, if you are so important that only your opinion or decision is vital for the functioning of the department, there is something fundamentally wrong with your local organisation. I always think it is insecurity from some control freaks. I also noticed that having a mobile ringing all the time gives the person a certain status; he or she is needed.

To stop this annoyance.

I think we should think about designing the lecture hall of the future where all wireless telecommunication connections are blocked automatically. Speaking of wireless connections, there is also a tendency to see people working on a computer during a lecture, mostly browsing the Internet for who knows what. Again, blocking the wireless Internet connections in the lecture hall would definitely be a good thing. So, do not let your attitude be influenced by the ill-mannered individuals and put your mobile on silent mode and do not play with your computer in a lecture hall. Just imagine you are the one giving the lecture, which took a lot of time to prepare, and everybody is busy doing other things rather than listening to you. This would be like, after the first words of your lecture, 30 people in the audience noisily opening a newspaper and starting to read.

6.2.2
Making Notes

Making notes is hardly ever necessary now. Most up-to-date medical meetings provide all lectures online after the meeting, not only the slides but also, more often than not, the audio; ever more frequently, this comes together with a video. The last is a no-frills video, which is shown together with the audio and slides on the Internet. Sometimes this service is free, sometimes one has to be a member of the host organisation to receive it, and sometimes one has to pay a little extra fee for this service. Always check with the organisation to find if they have this service available. Of course, there is always the abstract book, but you will learn that, for educational lectures, the abstract book does not always cover the contents of the presentation. Despite the fact that all material is readily available post-meeting in high quality, you still see people taking pictures of all the slides during a lecture or even filming the lecture. I have always found this irritating, and I hope you, as a novice, will never pick up this strange habit.

6.2.3
Asking Questions

Asking questions is something that you have to learn and to plan. I give you some basic rules here.

The first thing to learn and which has to be made absolutely clear is why you want to ask a question. The second thing is to let it be known what it is you are hoping to achieve by asking a question. Asking a question is often not "just" asking a question; it sometimes has a deeper meaning, a political or scientific dispute as background or even a personal vendetta. I give you a variety of reasons why a question is asked. Before you run to a microphone to ask your first question, please observe the people asking questions during your first few medical meetings and try to categorise them in one of these groups. This will help you a lot when you have the unstoppable urge to run to a microphone after a lecture. You will see that it is always the same notorious group who prominently "leads" the discussion. By the way, most experienced speakers know well how to handle this, and their answers are often either political or diplomatic. One should also realise that a speaker who just finished a completely unstructured and tangled lecture will not suddenly give a clear and structured answer to your question. In this case, any question is a waste of time unless one wants to demonstrate again the ignorance of the presenter.

It is my personal experience that approaching a speaker after a lecture to ask the speaker a question is often much more rewarding because he or she no longer feels the tension of being on the podium and therefore is more relaxed while answering your questions.

Of course, the culture of asking questions very much depends on the type of medical meeting you are attending. There are meetings where it is a habit or even a must to have "lively discussions" after every presentation; therefore, the presenters are ready and prepared. At this kind of meeting, there is ample time allocated in the programme for this. It is part of the culture or folklore or even the attraction of this specific meeting. Only when you are really ready will you go on stage to present your data. The advantage of this is that hardly any sloppy or half-finished data will be presented, which of course will contribute to the quality of the meeting. The downside of this is that juniors will often be put off making the leap to presenting as it seems intimidating, and the pool of presenters will therefore stay the same over many years, which will then prevent new, fresh and different scientific views coming forward. As is the case with all traditions, this is often hard to combat. I have no idea if any medical meeting holds a junior forum at which novice speakers can learn and practice (maybe even with a tutor) to become better prepared for the main stage. That would not be a bad idea.

I must say I still vividly remember my first question at a medical meeting. It was the second meeting I ever attended. It was probably a combination of my youthful enthusiasm and the open and inviting way the presenter gave the lecture that pushed me through my natural barrier. The presenter was a renowned U.S. radiologist speaking on treatment of renal artery stenosis; by the way, the presenter is still lecturing on this topic now, 23 years later. He talked about balloon angioplasty and his fantastic results with this technique in patients with renal artery obstructions. His lecture was clear and easy to understand, but during the lecture he made a side remark that caught my attention. He said that you had to blow up the dilatation balloon until it starts hurting. (Dilatation balloons were at that time still inflated with a syringe by hand.)
So, my obvious question after the lecture was what kind of pain would the patient feel and where would the patient feel it during the inflation of the dilatation balloon. He looked at me, seeing an obvious novice, and said "Not the patient, but until the syringe hurts in your hand". This brought an overwhelming bout of laughter from the audience and my first big lesson in lecture etiquette. Some question are better asked after the lecture in a one-on-one situation (by the way, I now know that the patient feels the pain in his flank).

6.3
Analysing Questions

If you really want to understand the social structure of a medical meeting, it is worthwhile to spend some time in understanding and analysing questions asked after a presentation. This can teach you a lot. In doing this, there is a certain resemblance to the modern discipline of ethology, which studies aspects of animal behaviour. I would certainly not dare to go as far as to compare a medical meeting with a monkey colony, but there are some remarkable similarities, and analysing questions is a great tool to show that.

Questions can be divided into several categories, but some fall into more than one. Classifying the questions is not only a great learning experience for those new to a medical meeting but also a nice game to play with colleagues after a lecture.

Group 1. This is the easiest and most straightforward question to score. It is also hoped to be the most common one.
- A question about something that was unclear during the lecture or not well presented
- A question that adds value to the lecture

Group 2. This question is sometimes more difficult.
- A question about something that was clearly explained during the lecture
- A question that shows that the person has been asleep, arrived late or is just a little bit stupid
- A question that already contains the answer

Group 3. Again, this is an easy question and often occurs.
- A question that is not related to the presented topic
- A question about a small detail (i.e. a p value on one slide)

Group 4. If you look for these questions, you will find them all the time.
- Not a question but a statement about something related to the lecture
- Some question or statement not even related to the lecture

So, now that you have categorised the questions, we can move up to the advanced level. This will give you good insight into the underlying politics of a meeting. You have to establish WHY the question was asked and WHAT the real meaning of the question was.

The WHY can be the following:
A. Because the questioner is interested in the answer.
B. Because the individual wants to help the presenter.
C. Because the questioner wants to show alpha dominance on this specific topic.
D. Because the individual is just a natural nuisance glued to any available microphone.
E. No one has a clue.

The WHAT can be
A. A presenter-friendly question
B. A presenter-hostile question
C. A question with no deeper meaning

Let us presume that someone just gave a great presentation about the difficult problems with angiotensin-converting enzyme (ACE) inhibitors in the African population with hypertension. After the presentation, any of following may be asked:

– *"Is there a problem with ACE-inhibitors in the African population?"*

This is a group 2 question with a sub-score of D or E and no further specification.

– *"Do you know anything about the Asian population, the topic of my research group?"*

This is a group 3 question with a sub-score of C plus D.

– *"We have studied a small African population with HIV, and our data do not support your presentation, dear colleague!"*

This is a group 4 question with a sub-score of E plus B.

The technique of how to answer questions is discussed elsewhere in this book (Sect. 4.12 of Chap. 4) as this is a permanent feature of your presentation for which you also have to prepare.

6.4
How to Avoid Annoying the Lecturer

The following is a summary of my top ten most encountered irritations during a lecture. These are to be avoided at all costs.

1. Snoring in the first few rows of the lecture hall
2. Coming late and then walking out before the lecture is finished
3. Answering your phone
4. Working on your computer during my lecture
5. Reading a newspaper
6. Talking to your neighbour throughout my lecture
7. Eating hot and smelly meals while I am lecturing
8. Not laughing at my pre-prepared jokes
9. Shaking your head in a "No, No" fashion all the time
10. Trying to seduce my beautiful junior assistant when I am giving a lecture

Please do not do this in any lecture hall, especially not when I am giving a lecture.

6.5 The Faculty

Every meeting needs some "great" names in its faculty to make the event more interesting for participants. I have learned over the years that great names are not always synonymous with great speakers and vice versa. Often, established and famous speakers at medical meetings place too much trust in their experience and are seen to repeat old lectures, with minor changes, for years. Generally, one can say that speakers in the circuit who speak at more than eight different medical meetings annually cannot be original at each of them. Of course, this is not true of all famous speakers. For the organisers of medical meetings, it is often difficult to bypass these "dinosaurs" as they bring with them a cloud of distinction that can add to the prestige of the meeting. You will see that meeting organisers sometimes try to sell a meeting based on these names. A "preliminary", sometimes called "invited", faculty is often a teaser in the first announcement of a meeting. It is not unusual for the final faculty to be much smaller, lacking the important names from the first announcement. Is this cheating? Well, it is, but we are living in a competitive world, and some advertisement is allowed.

Sometimes, a speaker is "hot" because he or she has just written a breakthrough paper or has published an important book. Often, however, it is not clear why other speakers are seen as hot or indispensable to the meeting. Maybe a vice-versa invitation policy might be an explanation.

A really bad habit of a number of meetings is to sell slots within their official programme to the industry partners to present the latest, or sometimes last year's, "scientific" news about their products or devices. This is misleading as the participants of the meeting are not made aware of the active industry participation. These company-sponsored presentations should always be separate from the main programme in clearly identifiable satellite symposia under the auspices of an independent programme committee. Moreover, the name of the sponsoring company should clearly appear next to the presentation.

6.6
Evaluation Forms

Another new thing that was not around some years ago are evaluation forms. Once the meeting was over and everybody had done his or her thing, we all went home and lived happily ever after – not anymore. In the early days of evaluations, we were asked to fill out evaluation forms at the end of a meeting, which the meeting organisers needed to give CME credits to the participants. Today, every last detail is evaluated – the meeting, the speakers, the chairpersons, the catering, the topics, the location – you name it, and it will be asked. Of course, this marketing evaluation is done to improve the quality of the next meeting, to lose bad speakers, to dump non-interesting topics and so on. This will improve the quality of your next meeting, so for your own good, hand in evaluation forms at as many symposia you attend if possible. Do not be shy or polite as these forms are always anonymous. Be blunt, tell the truth. If you think Doctor XY is a bad speaker and not somebody you want to see at a podium at your next medical meeting, just tell them. If many other fill out the forms the same, this poor presenter might even decide to read this book and make a glorious comeback.

Now that you know some basic principles of the social environment of a medical meeting, it is time to start preparing for your lecture. If you read and follow the instructions in the first part of this book, you will be fine.

Tips and Tricks

7

Contents

7.1
Getting Along with the Industry Partners

By now, you have given your excellent presentation, your PowerPoint was well received, and you are starting to feel relaxed. It is time for a further batch of important information. Remember, a medical meeting is a large social event with many players at all different levels. You want to celebrate your success, so you ask your colleagues if they want to join you for dinner that evening. However, much to your surprise, all your colleagues already have dinner plans for that evening and, by the way, for the next one. You are left behind in confusion. You should now proceed to the next paragraph.

We are always told that there is no such thing as a free lunch. Well, let me tell you something: There is. Although in many countries governments have introduced strict rules on what the industry can offer or do for physicians, a free lunch is still often possible. However, limousine pickup, five-star hotel rooms and a full side programme, sometimes even for the whole family (depending on your status and medical specialty), are no longer allowed in most countries. The consequences of ignoring such rules are serious, and most companies will not take the risk.

I was always told that the industry could afford this "investment" by charging higher prices for their products. I now very much doubt this as I have seen no price decreases since this extreme pampering of doctors has ceased. For a junior, stopping by the industry booth and having a cup of coffee while listening to a smart-talking sales rep is the first step to a five-course meal in a three-star restaurant. Before going to a meeting, always try to find out if your local salesperson will be there, and if not, find out who will be replacing this person. When your local rep visits your office before the meeting, talk to him or her about which "social events" will be happening at the upcoming meeting. Talk in detail about events you heard of through your colleagues. Let the salesperson know that you are

J.A. Reekers, *Presenting at Medical Meetings*,
DOI: 10.1007/978-3-642-12408-2_7, © Springer-Verlag Berlin Heidelberg 2010

aware of your colleagues' programme. Never ask to be taken out but make it natural or, indeed, unavoidable for them not to invite you. Even a professor or chief of a major department once started out as a junior. Early relations and growing together is vital for any company. Give them at least the impression that you are a potential high-flyer in (academic) medicine. If you are invited, do not immediately jump at the invitation; you have a full agenda, and you will let them know if the invitation will fit your schedule. As in many walks of life, it is not who or what you are, but who they think you are that counts.

Of course there are limits to how one should talk with the industry. Mutual respect is important. Remember that industry representatives are crucial to the existence of many meetings, and that they can often be an important source for new medical science. The following little anecdote is an example of very bad behaviour; nevertheless, I have seen in the past that the industry seems to have little power to stop this. Luckily, we now have improved and stricter regulations in most countries, which has made this kind of rudeness disappear.

Of course, the industry is not only there for the free lunch; they are, as mentioned, an extremely valuable source of knowledge. They can inform you on the latest products, upcoming trials and all kinds of background information. They can introduce you to important people. Remember, without them, there would be no meetings at all, regardless of size: They are the (financial) backbone of all scientific medical meetings. I therefore think they deserve respect, and you should always pay them this respect by visiting their booths. The technical exhibition is so important that at some meetings they require a separate entrance ticket for those not interested in the scientific programme. Working with the industry can bring you into contact with important investigators, and you might get the opportunity to join in on larger multi-centre trials, but take care to remain independent and not to become an industry frontman.

7.2
The Industry Frontman

What constitutes an industry frontman, how do you recognise him or her, and how do you deal with this person?
If you look in the dictionary for the word *frontman* you will find the following meaning:

- A man who serves as a nominal leader, but who lacks real authority.
- A person used as a cover for some questionable activity.

So, what is an industry frontman? This is somebody who is a spokesperson for promotional activities and for this uses an image based on artificial rather than real authority. One often sees them in their full glory as speakers of industry-sponsored satellite symposia. Let me be clear: Most speakers in industry-sponsored satellite symposia are genuinely excellent speakers, chosen for their academic reputation to speak about industry-related science. This is not a problem at all. These speakers speak from their own unbiased positions. A frontman, however, recites the words the industry wants to get across for promotional reasons. His or her air of being a renowned speaker is created without the backing of an authentic scientific curriculum vitae. This person can be used for many occasions, travels the world, but never pays a dollar out of his or her pocket. The frontman's reputation, however, can easily and quickly disappear into thin air. The person will then be removed from the scene with the same speed he or she was parachuted on to it. Beware of these false prophets.

7.3
Housing

Where to stay very much depends on your budget, your position in the medical hierarchy or your other local plans. If you are a junior with a low budget, it is sometimes not economical to book a hotel through the congress travel agent. You will probably pay top prices, even for three-star hotels. Unfortunately, searching for a hotel yourself during the time of the congress can be difficult as most of the larger meetings will have booked all available rooms. There is, however, a way to avoid this problem, a trick that I sometimes used in the past. Many travel agencies offer city tours; hotel rooms are prebooked long in advance and often come with fair-priced travel arrangements. They are not always close to the meeting place, but you could save a lot of money. Bed and breakfasts and shared holiday apartments (if the meeting is in a holiday destination) can also be an economical alternative to the four- and five-star congress hotels. I would generally avoid camping, park benches or sleeping on the beach. For more senior doctors, the four- and five-star hotels offered through the congress are more or less obligatory. Sharing a room with a colleague is an option but be sure the room has two separate beds unless you see this as an opportunity to be seized. "No honey, I was assured there would be two separate beds" is not the best opener for a lasting working relationship. Be aware that twin beds are most often two beds, but a twin-size bed is one large bed. Similarly, a double bed is one large bed and not double beds. If you really want to share, make sure you receive written confirmation from the hotel about the room category at the time of booking. If the meeting is in a hotel, the congress hotel is of course the most convenient.

7.4
Travelling

Most larger medical meetings are organised in places that are served by an international airport, so flying there is probably the easiest way to travel. Alternatives like carpooling and coming by train should be considered for the lower-budget traveller; however, budget airlines like EasyJet and Ryanair usually make these travel alternatives redundant when travelling within Europe. If you do travel with a budget airline, bear in mind that (as once happened to me) the taxi from the airport to the hotel can be more expensive than the flight. On the subject of taxis, if there is a large medical meeting in town and you look like a doctor, you are going to be charged an extortionate amount for a taxi ride. Some places in Europe are notorious for this, like Rome, Amsterdam and Athens. A straw hat and a camera around your neck might fool some taxi drivers but do not count on this. The best way to avoid this problem is to fix the price before you get in the taxi. Many airports have taxi booths where you can buy a taxi voucher; this is probably the best and most reasonable option.

Well, my dear colleagues this is the end of the book. Remember, this book is written from my personal experience and might therefore not always be applicable to your specific medical specialty or situation. Most of the information about how to present information comes from many sources, and the many books available in the field of marketing. I think selling a product is like "selling" medical information; it is the same mechanism. I hope that you will be a better presenter at your next meeting after reading this book, and I expect your future medical meetings to be more successful than ever before.

Yours sincerely,
Jim Reekers, MD